HEALTH PROMOTION AND HEALTH EDUCATION IN NURSING

Health Promotion and Health Education in Nursing

A FRAMEWORK FOR PRACTICE

Edited by

Dean Whitehead

and

Fiona Irvine

palgrave
macmillan

First published 2010 by
PALGRAVE MACMILLAN

Palgrave Macmillan in the UK is an imprint of Macmillan Publishers Limited,
registered in England, company number 785998, of Houndmills, Basingstoke,
Hampshire RG21 6XS.

Palgrave Macmillan in the US is a division of St Martin's Press LLC,
175 Fifth Avenue, New York, NY 10010.

Palgrave Macmillan is the global academic imprint of the above companies
and has companies and representatives throughout the world.

Palgrave® and Macmillan® are registered trademarks in the United States,
the United Kingdom, Europe and other countries.

ISBN 978–1–4039–4081–0

This book is printed on paper suitable for recycling and made from fully
managed and sustained forest sources. Logging, pulping and manufacturing
processes are expected to conform to the environmental regulations of the
country of origin.

A catalogue record for this book is available from the British Library.

10 9 8 7 6 5 4 3 2 1
19 18 17 16 15 14 13 12 11 10

Printed in China

Contents

Preface

Welcome to the first edition of this book, devoted to health promotion and health education for nurses working in health settings. Over the past decade or more, health service reform for many developed countries has witnessed radical shifts in the way that health care is delivered and resourced. Perhaps the most notable reform has been the shift from acute based primary, secondary and tertiary services to community and population health based services. Primary health care reform, underpinned by ideological and actual shifts in public health and health policy strategy, have relentlessly driven this reform. All of these activities come under the umbrella of *health promotion* in its current form. Many nurses (and other health professional groups, too) have struggled with this shift in health care provision. That said, and of late, there are more and more examples in nursing to draw from of a widening movement in line with broader health promotion strategy and shifts in health services and health policy. This has given rise to an increased awareness amongst nurses of the actual and potential impact of health promotion; and the growing recognition of the need truly to embrace health promotion in theory, practice and policy terms is encouraging. It is against this backdrop that the need for a book such as this proves timely.

There are a number of health promotion books in print, but there are very few that specifically target nurses and nursing practice. This book differs from most nursing titles in a number of ways. Rather than merely describing what health promotion is or is not, who does it and what it might look like (although this book does that, too), this book examines and describes the logical and practical process of how to incorporate health promotion as a framework for practice. The opening chapters are designed to set the scene for what health promotion (and health education) is, and how we contextualize it. Some later chapters build on this by noting and critiquing health promotion strategies at the national, international and global levels. In between, other chapters set the platform for identifying how health promotion can be incorporated into different nursing practice settings as a systematic process. It does the same for health education in its context as a sub-set of health promotion.

This book will appeal to all nurses and many other health professional groups who are interested in health promotion theory and who wish to engage, or are already engaged in, health promotion and health education practice and policy. At an educational level, this book will also appeal to, and serve well, the needs of most undergraduate and post-graduate programmes that contain papers and modules devoted to health promotion, health education, community and population health, and public health issues. We hope that you enjoy this book and gain from it as much as we have enjoyed the process of writing it.

DEAN WHITEHEAD
FIONA IRVINE

List of Figures and Tables

Figures

Tables

Acknowledgements

Dean and Fiona would like to extend thanks to all the individuals that contributed to this book. The commitment and enthusiasm of our colleagues in the UK and New Zealand ensured that the book chapters were completed on time and in keeping with the aims of the book. We are grateful to them all.

We also thank the team at Palgrave Macmillan for their help in turning the manuscript into a finished product. In particular, we thank Lynda Thompson and Kate Llewellyn for their support and encouragement throughout the process.

Finally, we would like to thank our families, colleagues and friends, whose support and tolerance throughout the process allowed us to focus on the book – which sometimes meant we were neglecting their needs.

Dean sends special thanks to Katie, Thomas, James and Joshua for their unstinting love and support – and also for allowing him the opportunity to be their personal bank manager and taxi driver. Fiona sends thanks to Stuart, Primrose and Amber for their continued understanding and encouragement.

The authors and publishers wish to thank the following for permission to use copyright material: Oxford University Press for Fig. 2.1, originally fig.6.1 (p. 102) in Downie, R. et al. (1996) *Health Promotion: Models and Values,* 2nd edn, Oxford: OUP; Taylor & Francis Books UK for Fig.2.2, originally fig.7.1 (p. 167) from Beattie, A. (1991) 'Knowledge and control in health promotion: a test case for social policy and theory' in Gage, J. et al. (eds) *The Sociology of the Health Service*, London: Routledge; Sage Publications Ltd for Fig.1.1 originally from Bracht, N. *et al.* (1999) *Health Promotion at the Community Level: New Advances*, Thousand Oaks, CA: Sage, and Fig. 2.3 originally from Caplan, R. and Holland, R. (1990) 'Rethinking health education theory', *Health Education Journal*, 49 (10–12); Nelson Thornes Ltd for Fig. 2.4, originally fig.1.7 in Tones, K. and Tilford, S. (2001) *Health Promotion: Effectiveness, Efficiency and Equity*, 3rd edn, Cheltenham: Nelson Thornes; Pearson Education, Inc. for Fig. 2.5 from Pender, N.J. *et al.* (2006) *Health Promotion in Nursing Practice*, New Jersey: Pearson Prentice Hall; McGraw Hill Education for Fig. 4.1 from Green, L.W. and Kreuter, M.W. (1999) *Health Promotion Planning*, Palo Alto, CA: Mayfield. Every effort has been made to trace all the copyright-holders, but if any have been inadvertently overlooked the publishers will be pleased to make the necessary arrangement at the first opportunity.

Notes on the Contributors

Caroline Bradbury-Jones, PhD, MA, BSc, RGN, RM, HV
Caroline is Lecturer in Nursing at Bangor University in Wales. Caroline qualified as a nurse in 1983, and then as a midwife in 1988. Following this, she practised as a health visitor for ten years in both rural and urban communities in the UK. During this time, she developed a keen interest in the public health and health promotion aspect of the role. She was involved in several important community initiatives relating to prevention of postnatal depression, child protection, and the promotion of health in ethnic minority populations. Since moving into nurse education in 2001, she has retained an active interest in health promotion, and teaches this topic on undergraduate and postgraduate programmes.

Ruth Cross, MSc, BSc(Hons), PGCHE, RN
Ruth is Senior Lecturer in Public Health and Health Promotion at Leeds Metropolitan University, with a background in adult health nursing. She has wide experience in health, health care services and health provision, both in the UK and in Sub-Saharan Africa. She lectures on public health and health promotion across a wide range of undergraduate and postgraduate courses.

Fiona Irvine, PhD, MSc, RN
Fiona is Professor of Nursing at Liverpool John Moores University. Her clinical background is in community nursing. She worked as a district nurse and a Macmillan nurse, before moving into nurse education and nursing research. Fiona has secured research funding from a number of sources in order to undertake research studies that relate to language and cultural awareness. Fiona's research interests also extend to health promotion and community nursing, and she works closely with primary health care professionals on practice related research. Fiona is co-director of LLAIS, the Language Awareness Infrastructure Support Service that, as part of CRC Cymru, provides advice, support and a research lead to Thematic Research Networks across Wales about Welsh language awareness in health and social care. She is thematic coordinator for the organization and delivery of services theme of the Institute of Health Research at Liverpool John Moores University. Fiona has published numerous journal articles and book chapters relating to her research work.

Sean Mackay, MHSc, BNurs(Hons), PGCHE, RGN, RHV, NMC, FHEA
Sean is Head of Public Health and Primary Care at Liverpool John Moores University. He manages programmes in community and public health nursing, and teaches health promotion on a variety of programmes. He leads an annual public health field trip to the Gambia. Sean supported the training of peer educators in sexual health in Indonesia as part of a DFID funded project, and has taught in Ethiopia, Finland and Malaysia.

Sue McAndrew, PhD, MSc, BSc (Hons), CPN Cert., RMN
Sue is Lecturer at the University of Leeds. Sue leads the graduate pre-registration
nursing programme (mental health) and continues to work actively in primary
mental health care, dealing with a number of community based health promotion
initiatives. Her main interests are in psychoanalytic and managerial discourse, in
which areas she has published widely.

Rod Thomson, MEd, MSc, Dip Ad Ed, Dip HV, RMN, RGN, RHV, FRCN,
FFP
Rod is Consultant in Public Health (Community Safety) for Sefton Primary Care
Trust in Merseyside and Honorary Professor at Liverpool John Moores University.
His current role includes lead responsibility for Health Protection and Emergency
Planning/Response. Rod's nursing career spans primary care, mental health and
accident/emergency nursing. He has worked in various parts of the UK, but has
been based in the North West of England since 1991. Rod is an active member of
the Royal College of Nursing and has held several national posts, including Chair of
the Health Visitors Forum and Vice Chair of the Nurses in Executive and Strategic
Roles Forum. He is currently Vice Chair of the RCN Congress for the College's
annual conference and CPD event. In 2002, he received the Royal College of Nursing's highest award – a fellowship – in recognition of an exceptional contribution to
the art and science of nursing. He is also a Fellow of the Faculty of Public Health
(UK). Rod's nursing and public health links have taken him as far afield as Australia,
Canada, Cuba, Japan, Taiwan and the USA, as well as many parts of Europe. Rod is
also a steering group member of the International Council of Nurses Disaster
Preparedness Network.

Tony Warne, PhD, MBA, RMN, JP
Tony is Professor in Mental Health Care, Head of School of Nursing and Associate
Dean for the Research Faculty of Health and Social Care at the University of Salford.
The focus of his research interest is on inter-personal, intra-personal and extra-
personal relationships, using a psychodynamic and managerialist analytical discourse.
This research has centred on exploring the impact of such relationships on nursing
practice, policy, organization and, particularly, nurse education and the preparation
for practice. He has published extensively and is the co-editor and author of the
book *Using Patient Experience in Nurse Education* and *Creative Approaches to
Health and Social Care Education*. He is the Associate Editor of the *International
Journal of Mental Health Nursing*. Tony has been a Magistrate for the past 14 years,
where his main interest lies in issues related to young offenders.

Dean Whitehead, PhD, MSc, BEd, RN
Dean is Senior Lecturer in the School of Health and Social Services at Massey
University in New Zealand, having emigrated from the UK in 2004. Dean is a
prolific researcher and publisher, where the main focus lies with his research interests in health promotion and health education theory and practice, health policy,
public health and primary health care, with over 100 theoretical/research and book
publications in these fields. Dean sits on several international executive editorial/
advisory journal boards, including the *Journal of Clinical Nursing* and

Nurse Education Today. He also has extensive experience of reviewing and advising for over 20 journal review panels, involving a number of leading international nursing journals, but also including journals such as *Health Promotion International, Health Education, Health Education Research, Global Health Promotion, Health Policy* and *Preventative Medicine*. Dean's current national research focus lies with several New Zealand based health promotion projects that are investigating the assessment of both childhood nutrition and bullying issues, as they relate to the World Health Organization's Health-Promoting Schools network. His PhD was an epistemology of health promotion as it related to clinical theory, policy and practice issues.

Key Features

The list below outlines the key features of each chapter, and how they are meant to be used:

Objectives
The main aims of the chapter, to help you plan your reading

Key terms
The central concepts of the chapter, to act as a quick reference

Tutorial briefs
Set exercises designed to support your learning

Summary points
Short lists of the main arguments to aid revision

Health Promotion in Action boxes
Examples of health promotion studies and projects and their main findings, to help you link the theory to primary clinical practice

Additional points
Manageable, bite-sized pieces of information, to illuminate the chapter content

Additional resources
Print and online sources to help you further research the material covered in the book

All additional pedagogy has been designed to help you interact with the text, and to help you better understand the main points presented.

Note that the Tutorial Brief Answers can be found at the back of the book on pages 183–98.

CHAPTER 1

Contextualizing Health Promotion

Fiona Irvine

Objectives

By the end of this chapter you should be able to:

- Discuss the main dimensions of health
- Explore the similarities and differences between health education, health promotion and public health
- Examine the main attributes of health education, health promotion and public health
- Justify the use of health education and health promotion approaches in nursing

---

Key terms

- Empowerment
- Health education
- Health promotion
- Public health
- Socio-political change

Introduction

'Health promotion' is now a well-established term, the strength of which lies in the fact that it is multidisciplinary – cutting across professional disciplines and drawing inspiration from a wide theoretical base. However, the eclectic nature of health promotion can often result in a lack of clarity about the meaning of the concept. Thus, it is well recognized that the term 'health promotion' can be ambiguous (Tones and Tilford 2001). Since the underpinning theory of health promotion

1

emerges from a number of subject areas, it is no surprise that nurses can find it difficult to product a clear-cut definition of health promotion. Indeed, Tones and
Tilford (1994: 2) believe that health promotion:

> means all things to all people – who are united only in their agreement that it is
> rather desirable.

Added to the confusion about health promotion is the fact that it can be hard to
differentiate between 'health education', 'health promotion' and 'public health'.
Often, these terms are used interchangeably or to mean different things (Whitehead
2004; Earle 2007).

Whitehead (2004) contends that the paradigms of health education and health
promotion might be closely related, but they are not inter-dependent. He separates
the terms from one another – arguing that health promotion has developed in shape
and focus, and that it is now possible to explore the paradigms of health education
and health promotion in their own right. Moreover, a number of authors (Webster and
French 2002; Scott-Samuel and Springett 2007) argue that public health and health
promotion should be viewed as separate, but overlapping, domains.

The purpose of this chapter is to clarify the meaning of the terms 'health education', 'health promotion' and 'public health' as separate entities; to explore the
relationship between the concepts; and to discuss the characteristics that distinguish
them. It will give an exploration of the concepts to clarify their meaning and help
prevent nurses from using the terms ambiguously and interchangeably. However,
before we can start to explore these concepts, for which health is the core, we need
to clarify our comprehension of health itself.

What is health?

An exploration of health education, health promotion and public health is predicated on an understanding of health. Health is a challenging concept to define as it
means different things to different people, and our understanding of health is influenced by cultural, socio-economic and personal contexts (Seedhouse 2001; Scott-
Samuel and Springett 2007). Writers, practitioners and individuals hold notions of
health as a commodity, health as an ideal state, health as the ability to function
normally and health as a basis for adaption. Seedhouse (2001) gives a full exploration and critique of these theories of health and, in so doing, demonstrates that each
perspective has its limitations. He puts forward the notion that health is equivalent
to a set of conditions that enable individuals to achieve their realistic, chosen and
biological potential – and recognizes that the importance of these conditions
depends on the individual context. In other words, he sees health as a flexible
concept and the level of health that an individual holds varies depending on circumstances.

Seedhouse's notion of health is in agreement with that put forward by the *Ottawa
Charter for Health Promotion* (WHO 1986). The *Ottawa Charter* was the product
of the first international conference on health promotion and is considered to be

highly influential in shaping health promotion from then to today. It portrays health as a resource for everyday life rather than merely the objective of living. In this case, Weare (2002) argues that free choice has to be at the centre of the concept of health, since it becomes a resource to enable individuals and communities to function in the way that *they* find acceptable. Thus, according to Seedhouse (2001), health has to be viewed as a 'fuzzy' concept, as it is given its definition by the inherently different social and personal context.

 Tutorial brief 1.1

Think about the term 'health'. List the main things that would allow you to classify yourself as healthy.

What influences health?

It is accepted that a number of social, biological, behavioural, environmental and economic factors influence health. Dahlgren and Whitehead's (1991) much cited model demonstrates that the determinants of health are tied up with individual lifestyle factors; social and community networks; living and working conditions; and general socio-economic, cultural and environmental conditions. Similarly, Tones and Tilford (2001) present a model that focuses on the *macro* (large), *meso* (middle) and *micro* (small) influences on health. The general consensus is that the factors that influence health do not work in isolation; rather, they involve a complex web of interaction. The case of obesity provides an example of how determinants interact.

The prevalence of obesity in Western society has risen significantly over the past few decades and there is clear evidence that obesity gives rise to ill health. Obesity has been shown to cause high blood pressure, heart disease, type-2 diabetes mellitus and various cancers (Reidpath et al. 2002). In short, obesity is shown to lessen life expectancy markedly. It is clear that various factors are associated with obesity. In relation to lifestyle, dietary factors such as limited consumption of fruit and vegetable as well as high fat and sugar intake have been shown to lead to obesity. Moreover, a sedentary lifestyle is associated with being overweight and having a high body saturated fat percentage. There is evidence also of obesity being associated with causal genes (Rankinen et al. 2006). However, a genetic predisposition does not invariably lead to obesity, and lifestyle factors are not always down to individual choice. Socio-economic factors such as family and peer group behaviour and socio-economic status (SES) are known to have direct influence on levels of obesity. For example, Reidpath et al. (2002) demonstrate that as SES declines, the risk of obesity increases. One explanation put forward for this is the tendency for the poor, perhaps out of necessity, to eat cheaper processed energy-dense foods.

Living and working conditions also have an effect on dietary intake and obesity. For example, the notion of the obesogenic environment (namely, an environment that encourages the consumption of food and/or discourages physical activity) is now well recognized. In effect, an environmentally induced change in energy balance results in an increased risk of obesity. In turn, political, social and economic forces shape the conditions in which people live. A case-in-point is the proliferation of fast food outlets, which enable access to relatively cheap, high energy, high fat foods. The irony of this is that these outlets have flourished because of the political and economic environment that has encouraged the growth of fast food companies – which evidently make a positive contribution to the overall economic climate and help to improve standards of living. Thus, we can see the complex interaction that takes place between the *macro*, political and economic factors; the *meso*, community-related factors; and the *micro*, individual factors that have led to the obesity epidemic (Tones and Tilford 2001).

Inequalities in health

A major concern for health promotion is that, although overall the health of the population is improving and people are living longer, health inequalities are ever widespread and the health status of different groups varies considerably. In Chapter 8, a detailed account is given of the different patterns of global health *between* populations. Here, this section will consider differences *within* populations.

Sociological factors including social class, poverty, gender and race directly influence health status. In the 1970s, some 30 years after the development of the welfare state and the establishment of the National Health Service (NHS) in the United Kingdom (UK), a growing concern about the gap in health status between the social classes led to the establishment of a government working-group and the subsequent publication of the Black Report (DHSS 1980). The Black Report showed a clear relationship between occupational class and morbidity and mortality. For almost every type of illness and disability that was investigated, a positive association between social class and health status was shown, whereby those in higher social classes were far less likely to suffer from illness or disability and more likely to live longer than their counterparts in lower social classes. The Report also gave evidence of other variations in health status. It showed regional variations (North versus South divide) in health, gender differences (usually more marked in men than women) in patterns of health, and higher incidence of a range of diseases (such as heart disease) amongst individuals from ethnic minority groups. Since the Report, societal changes (such as the advent of 'girl power') have adjusted and changed health status between different members of the population. Young females today, within a more liberal social environment, are more likely to adopt high-risk lifestyle choices than previously. In the twenty-first century, the existence of social inequalities in health, in the UK, is not disputed and striking differences between groups persist. However, this is not just a feature of UK society. In 2005 the Commission on Social Determinants of Health (CSDH) was set up by the World Health Organization (WHO) to marshal the evidence on what can be done to promote health equity and to foster a global movement to achieve it. Its recent report on the social determinants of health offers compelling evidence to

Table 1.1 Evidence of health inequalities within populations

Race	Life expectancy at birth (LEB) among indigenous Australians is substantially lower (59.4 for males and 64.8 for females in the period 1996–2001) than that of all Australians (76.6 and 82.0, respectively, for the period 1998–2000) (Aboriginal and Torres Strait Islander Social Justice Commissioner 2005).
Gender	Women's lower status in South Asia is the strongest contributor to child malnutrition in that region (Smith and Haddad 2000).
Social class	In Europe, the increased risk of dying among middle-aged adults in the lowest socio-economic groups ranges from 25 per cent to 50 per cent, and even 150 per cent (Mackenbach 2005).

demonstrate the continued existence of health inequalities within populations (CSDH 2008). It states that:

> In countries at all levels of income, health and illness follow a social gradient: the lower the socioeconomic position, the worse the health.

There is abundant evidence from around the world to uphold the position that inequalities in health related to race, gender and SES exist and have a major impact on the health status of individuals and communities. CSDH (2008) cites a number of examples of such inequalities, as shown in Table 1.1.

This stark evidence of health inequalities leads the CSDH (2008: 1) to state that:

> This unequal distribution of health-damaging experiences is not in any sense a 'natural' phenomenon but is the result of a toxic combination of poor social policies and programmes, unfair economic arrangements, and bad politics.

If health inequality is not a natural phenomenon, but one that global society has created, then it follows that action can be taken to tackle inequalities and bring about health equity. Nurses, who form a sizeable professional group (the largest by far of health professionals) within global health services, have an important contribution to make in tackling these issues. To promote health effectively, nurses need to understand how determinants of health interact, why inequalities exist and what measures can be taken to bring about changes to these factors to affect health in a positive way. Thus, they need to define their health-promoting work and establish systematic processes for their practice (see Chapter 4).

Differentiating the concepts of health education, health promotion and public health

It is important to make a conceptual distinction between health education, health promotion and public health in order to allow a clear foundation from which nurses can define their work, and identify and evaluate their roles. Douglas (2007) provides a useful distinction between individual and structuralist approaches to health promotion, suggesting that individual approaches focus on encouraging and empowering people to change their behaviour and adopt a healthy lifestyle, whereas structuralist approaches focus on efforts to change the wider determinants of health – such as the physical, social and economic environment. Douglas (2007) also acknowledges that some health protection approaches – such as the provision of immunization or screening – lay between individual and structuralist approaches, since they require an element of change on the part of both the individual and service provision.

Health promotion has many different interpretations and perspectives. It refers to a set of principles that rely on particular underlying values as well as describing ways of working. Central to contemporary health promotion practice is an emphasis on social action, tackling the determinants of health and addressing key issues such as inequalities in health and disempowerment. The purpose is, therefore, to make a difference to the causes of ill health rather than simply focusing on the consequences of it. This can be a challenge for nurses, many of whom face the consequences of ill health in their daily practice and whose work priorities might constrain them from focusing on the causes of ill health. Writers, such as Tones and Green (2004), believe that health education is tied up with activities that are designed to facilitate health related learning and, ultimately, lifestyle or behaviour change for people. To some extent, then, it is concerned with helping people to help themselves – an approach that sits comfortably in nursing.

Public health in its most simplistic form refers to the health of a population. However, there are various interpretations of public health that identify its different priorities and approaches. For some, public health is an umbrella term referring to all activities aimed at improving the health of the public, to which health promotion makes a major contribution (Macdonald and Bunton 2002). For others, public health is synonymous with a medical model and is concerned with preventive medicine, which focuses on measuring, controlling and preventing illness and disease (Scott-Samuel and Springett 2007). Because of these conflicting perspectives, it is not possible to give an authoritative definition of public health. The examination of health education, health promotion and public health by various authors helps to offer some distinction between the three concepts. This chapter now moves on to offer a more detailed exploration of each.

Summary point

Health promotion falls into the structuralist approach discussed earlier. Health education is concerned with the individual approach, and public health sits between the two approaches.

Health education

One way of identifying the distinguishing features of health education is to consider it as a process – how the service operates, and an outcome – what the service produces. In the case of health education, the process entails the imparting of health related information; the outcome involves influencing the knowledge and attitudes of individuals, empowering individuals and, ultimately, bringing about behavioural change and subsequent improved health.

Health education as information-giving

From the many definitions of health education that are found in the literature, it is evident that health education is tied up with information-giving. However, while this might sound simplistic, information-giving in health education is a complex process. It moves beyond imparting information and advice, to developing a cooperative process between the professional and the client; this involves clarifying values, exploring attitudes, motivational techniques and enabling processes (Sidell 2000; Tones and Tilford 2001). Health education focuses on change at the individual level, but can take the form of group work or mass media campaigns to reach the individual (Whitehead 2000). The health educator uses communication, together with educational and counselling methods, to motivate individuals and groups to bring about health related change. When effective, individual approaches can help to reduce people's risk of ill health but the nature of the intervention, normally with individuals or small groups, means that the effect on the total population is limited.

Health education as self-empowerment

There is a growing body of literature arguing that empowerment is a desirable outcome of health education (Tones and Green 2004), where the goal is to encourage personal growth through the enhancement of self-esteem and assertiveness (Sidell 2000). However, the discussion of empowerment can lead to some confusion when trying to distinguish between health promotion and health education. For example, Whitehead (2004) identifies empowerment as an element of progressive *health education*, whereas Rissel (1994) believes that empowerment embodies the basis (*raison d'être*) of health promotion. Rissel's (1994) contention – that two forms of empowerment exist; namely, *self-empowerment* and *community-empowerment* – helps to clarify how empowerment relates to both health education and health promotion. Gibson (1991: 359) defines self-empowerment, as:

> the social process of recognizing, promoting and enhancing people's ability to meet their own needs, solve their own problems and mobilize the necessary resources in order to feel in control of their own lives.

Self-empowerment requires *intrapersonal* aspects – such as the development of self-esteem and self-efficacy, and the enhancement of decision-making abilities. It also contains an *interpersonal* component, involving sharing, helping and partnerships that enable people to make autonomous decisions about their health.

According to the *Ottawa Charter for Health Promotion*, empowerment enables people to take control over their own lives and health status (WHO 1986). It is evident that the WHO's form of self-empowerment centres on people's ability to develop skills, understanding and awareness. This, in turn, facilitates individuals to

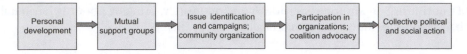

Figure 1.1 The empowerment continuum
Source: Bracht et al. (1999).

use personal resources to maximize their chances of developing healthy lifestyles and is more consistent with the concept of health education (Laverack 2007).

Bracht et al. (1999) identify empowerment as a continuum and this helps to further distinguish the relationship of empowerment to health education and health promotion (see Figure 1.1). Bracht and colleagues suggest that empowerment, at the individual (health education) level, involves personal development – advancing into empowerment at the structural (health promotion) level, where coalitions are developed to bring about political and social action.

Rissel (1994) views empowerment at the community or structural level, where a macro component exists, as community empowerment. He interprets community empowerment as self-empowerment 'plus', where social and political action is taken for the redistribution of resources in favour of the community in question. From the discussions so far, it is evident that community empowerment is viewed as a discrete attribute of *health promotion* and I will return to this later in the chapter.

Skelton (1994) is sceptical of the reasons for signing up to an ethos of empowerment. He believes that many professionals use the term 'empowerment' when, in reality, they are adopting a strategy that is essentially based on coercing clients to engage in behaviours that are advocated by the health educators. This is an approach that is labelled by Laverack (2007) as 'power-over'. MacDonald (1998) mirrors this. He replaces the term empowerment with *impowerment*; this is where power is conferred on clients by someone in authority – that is, health professionals.

A key theme for nurses is the authority that they hold that enables them to empower their clients. Nurses work in bureaucratic and hierarchical systems that are characteristically disempowering and, consequently, they can lack autonomy and control. If nurses have no power to relinquish, then they are in no position to empower others. Someone can only possess a certain amount of power if another person loses an equivalent amount. However, this position is dismissed by authors such as Laverack (2005), who contends that empowerment does not involve bestowing power; rather, it is an enabling process that involves an interpersonal dimension of sharing resources, helping each other and developing constructive relationships. This approach to empowerment is identified as 'power-with' – one in which nurses can readily engage (Laverack 2007).

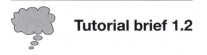 **Tutorial brief 1.2**

Identify the types of power that are relevant to you and your clients in your practice. To what extent might they prevent/promote health education and health promotion practices?

Dilemmas that relate to the relationship between power and empowerment are clearly pertinent for nurses. Whitehead (2004) claims that nurses are making some advances in the promotion of individuals' health through empowerment. It is clear from the literature that empowerment is seen as a positive concept that is intuitively appealing and a desirable outcome of health education (Sidell 2000). However, it is also fair to say that empowerment is not the desired *ultimate* outcome of health education but, rather, a means of ensuring that individuals develop the knowledge, attitudes, personal skills and self-esteem to be able to adopt a lifestyle that is conducive to good health. This leads to another key attribute of health education – that of behavioural change.

Health education as behaviour-change

There is considerable evidence available that demonstrates that lifestyle behaviour influences health (Kemm 2003). The justification underpinning this body of evidence is based on the fact that, since the 1970s, in Western society people have mainly died of diseases of affluence. These diseases include coronary heart disease, cerebro-vascular disease, chronic obstructive pulmonary disease and strokes – which are principally caused by unhealthy lifestyles (see Chapter 8 for greater detail on morbidity rates at a global level). McQueen (1987) identifies four critical behaviours that adversely affect health: smoking, sedentary lifestyle, poor nutrition and alcohol misuse. He ascribes these to a group that he labels the 'Holy Four'. More than twenty years on from McQueen's (1987) observations, the magnitude of the 'Holy Four' is still in evidence, with recent research demonstrating that avoiding smoking, engaging in physical activity, consuming only moderate amounts of alcohol, and a healthy diet can add up to fourteen years to people's life expectancy (BBC 2008). Bennett and Murphy (1997) add high-risk sexual activity to this list – a behaviour that has emerged as a significant contributory force to morbidity and mortality rates since the early 1980s, especially linked to HIV/AIDS in sub-Saharan Africa.

One way of addressing the increased morbidity and mortality rates associated with potentially harmful health-related behaviours is to adopt a behaviour-change approach to health education. Tones and Tilford (1994: 14) define such an approach as:

the persuasion of individuals to adopt behaviours believed to reduce the risk of disease.

The literature is full of accounts of interventions that aim to help and support individuals to alter their risky behaviour – either before or after the onset of illness, disease or disability. A cursory exploration of recent health education publications provides details of smoking cessation interventions in Northern Ireland (Thompson et al. 2007), weight-loss support in Greece (Georgiadis et al. 2006), a healthy-eating and physical-activity project in New Zealand (Williden et al. 2006) and anti-drug interventions in France (Peretti-Watel 2005). All these studies use structured and theoretically-informed strategies, designed to work with target groups to bring about a change in behaviour. They report varying levels of success.

Health promotion in action

Thompson et al. (2007) evaluated the success of a community nurse-led smoking cessation clinic – conducted in one National Health Service Trust in Northern Ireland. The clinic operated a group therapy approach. The study employed quantitative and qualitative methods of data collection. The authors found that the smoking cessation clinic helped 29.2 per cent of those who registered at the clinic to quit smoking at the end of the six-week course. Results indicated that participants had gained motivation from the 'group' experience, from the lowering of their carbon monoxide readings and from the positive attitude of the smoking cessation support nurses. However, the six-month follow-up suggested that a number of those who had given up smoking had relapsed into their previous smoking habit.

Given the evidence that demonstrates the link between lifestyle and ill health, it might seem appropriate that behavioural-change approaches have a significant position in health education. Indeed, according to Caraher (1994), nurses make behavioural-change approaches the mainstay of their health related work. More recently, Irvine (2007) and Casey (2007) both demonstrate that nurses continue to adopt strategies that focus on lifestyle risk factors. Widespread adoption of this approach essentially perpetuates the ethos that individuals are responsible for their own health. However, the position and impact of behavioural-change approaches in health education is contested, because changing a client's health related behaviour is notoriously problematic and, as argued earlier in this chapter, individual behaviour is not the primary determinant of health. At worst, the lifestyle and behaviour-change approach is considered by some to be unethical because it gives rise to 'victim-blaming'– where people are made to feel responsible and culpable for any developing ill health status (Tones and Green 2004). In this context, a behavioural-change approach is arguably one that is best avoided. However, behaviour-change should not be totally dismissed by nurses, as it can be reasonable to expect behavioural change in individuals – if careful consideration is given to the underpinning theoretical and practical constructs (Whitehead and Russell 2004).

Summary point

The attributes of health education can be categorized into those that relate to the process and those that relate to the outcome. The focus of health education generally is on the individual.

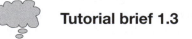

Tutorial brief 1.3

Can you identify the main elements of health education? Write a list of their main strengths and limitations that could affect your health-related work.

Making health education effective

In order to be effective health educators, nurses need a sound knowledge of what is meant by 'health education'. They should be conversant with the underlying principles of health education and knowledgeable of the various processes that can be effectively adopted to educate for health – as well as the outcomes that should realistically be expected when adopting a health education approach. For instance, the recipient of health education needs to be ready to receive health advice, and they must have the ability to assimilate it and to act on that advice to change or modify their behaviour (Whitehead 2004). Other factors – such as resources, time, support of colleagues and a personal commitment to health education – will also need to be present to enable nurses to engage effectively in health education.

Consequences of health education

Ultimately, health education should lead to the improvement of the health of individuals. However, it is likely that this aim will be achieved incrementally and will be determined by the outcomes of health education related to knowledge gain, awareness-raising, individual empowerment and behavioural change. While it is clear that health education now stands as a discrete concept, it nevertheless, makes a significant contribution to health promotion (Rawson 2002; Tones and Green 2004). Indeed, Kemm (2003) argues that an educational element features in nearly all health promotion activities. Knowing this, it is possible to move on to the distinct concept of health promotion.

 Tutorial brief 1.4

Think of a health education campaign or programme in which nurses are most likely to be involved. Identify, in increments, the consequences of the intervention that you could expect.

Summary point

Health education can be viewed as a process and an outcome. The process entails informing individuals about health and illness, and the risks and benefits associated with unhealthy and healthy lifestyles. The outcomes of health education are self-empowerment and behavioural change to embrace a healthy lifestyle. Health education requires effort on the part of the individual and the health educator. The consequence of health education is the improvement of the health of individuals.

Health promotion

Definitions of health promotion are diverse and represent many different conceptualizations of health. The *Ottawa Charter* (WHO 1986) sees improving health as the
outcome of health promotion and the various measures put in place to enable people
to increase control over their health as the process. The values underpinning the
health promotion process are participation, enablement and empowerment, equity
and social justice (Scott-Samuel and Springett 2007). These values represent a
progressive notion of health promotion involving processes that seek to address the
wider determinants of health as part of community development and collective
social action.

Health promotion as community development

Community development is highly regarded in the health promotion literature. For
example, Labonte and Robertson (1996) believe that community development is
the best strategy for remedying underlying social determinants of health – such as
economic, fiscal, political, environmental and ecological issues. This contention is
supported by a number of authors, who identify community development as the
most 'authentic' or ideal form of health promotion (Rawson 2002) and 'central' to
health promotion (Tones and Green 2004). In the health promotion literature,
there appear to be two main orders of community development. The first centres on
what Labonte and Robertson (1996) refer to as a 'community-based' approach.
Here, a lead agency mobilizes the local community to work in collaboration on a
disease-specific or behaviour-orientated issue (Mittlemark 1999). Labonte and
Robertson (1996) indicate that, when this approach is adopted, the health problem
is identified by the mobilizing agency. There are many examples of this type of
work, focusing on issues such as smoking (Ritchie et al. 2004), young people and
alcohol (Huckle et al. 2005) and classic coronary heart disease programmes, such as
the North Karelia Project in Finland (Puska 1995). Community empowerment
programme activities normally involve agendas that are pre-determined by health
promotion professionals and include strategies such as involvement of the public in
task forces, mass media campaigns, health fairs and public events.

The community-based approach to health promotion is subject to some criticism. For example, approaches that are based on disease or a lifestyle orientation
often have little reference to one another and can lead to omission or duplication of
efforts in reaching individuals (Berentson-Shaw and Price 2007). Moreover, focusing on measurable objectives and risk factor targets in community-based health
promotion can trivialize some problems and overlook others. Jensen (1997)
contends that community-based health promotion often fails to consider the wider
social and economic issues that are normal social determinants of people's health.
What are health priorities to health service agencies might well not reflect the health
priorities of the communities themselves. This type of community-based activity
bears close resemblance to health education; the difference being that one is at the
individual level, while the other targets the whole community.

Pelletier et al. (1997) claim that 'true' community development aims to empower the community, and that the decision-making processes that relate to the objectives and activities of a strategy are owned by that community. Thus, it enables communities to identify problems, develop solutions and facilitate change. In other words, community development is user-led and, as such, demands innovative ways of working that challenge the traditional medical or behavioural-change approaches (see Chapter 2 for greater detail on the different approaches to health education and health promotion). Asked to identify its main health priorities, most communities will not rank highly lifestyle-related behavioural programmes (for example, smoking cessation). Instead, they will often target issues centred on crime, justice, policing, pollution, welfare, transport, housing and so on. Based on the work of Henderson and Thomas (1980), Tones and Green (2004) outline key steps and stages in the community development process, which involve:

- Planning and negotiating entry
- Getting to know the community
- Working out what to do next
- Making contacts and bringing people together
- Forming and building organizations
- Helping the community to clarify goals and priorities
- Keeping organization going
- Dealing with friends and enemies
- Leavings and endings.

Adopting the community development approach means that an interactive dialogue takes place in a community and that action takes place across the community as a whole, with professionals sharing authority and responsibility with the community (Mittlemark 1999).

Health promotion in action

Ritchie et al.'s (2004) study evaluated the effect of a community-based approach to health promotion entitled 'Breathing Space'. The initiative aimed to produce a significant shift in community norms towards non-toleration and non-practice of smoking in a low-income area in Edinburgh, Scotland. The authors used a quasi-experimental design, which incorporated a process evaluation in order to provide a description of the development and implementation of the intervention. Drawing on qualitative data from the process evaluation, their paper explored the varied, and sometimes competing, understandings of the endeavour held by those implementing the intervention. The data illustrate how different understandings of community development had implications for the joint planning and implementation of Breathing Space objectives. In addition, they show that the varied understandings raise questions about the appropriateness and viability of utilizing community development approaches in the context of a behaviour-orientated issue such as smoking.

Health promotion as community empowerment

The previous discussions assist in demonstrating that community development is the desirable *process* of health promotion and is the means by which the expected *outcome* of community empowerment is reached (Bracht et al. 1999). Mittlemark (1999) defines community empowerment as communities making choices and becoming involved in the political processes that affect their lives. A similar position is taken by Laverack (2007), who believes that community empowerment entails communities gaining more control over the decisions and resources that influence their lives – and this includes the determinants of health and well-being status. Therefore, Laverack (2007) argues that health promotion involves a redistribution of power so that health professionals act as the facilitators of community participation, community action and, ultimately, community empowerment.

Community empowerment, however, is not without its limitations, which feature in a similar vein to the criticisms directed at self-empowerment. The issue of the agenda of health promoters is of relevance here. Difficulties can exist because of the discrete community dynamics that manifest in community development work. The loyalties of health promoters are often to their organization, rather than to the community. Thus, problems can develop because of the different health rationales and priorities that exist between communities and health promotion agencies. This problem however, is not insurmountable. As Lazenbatt et al. (2000) demonstrate in their study, nurses are engaging in community development work that identifies health needs, targets health and social needs through health promotion, addresses the structural factors that affect health and establishes social support networks. They demonstrate that careful selection of community development workers, who have personal allegiances to the community, will serve to avert the problems that arise because of different understandings of life processes within that community. Nevertheless, with these measures in place, the question of power is still likely to surface in community development work.

Authors, such as Dixon and Sindall (1994), contest that lip service is often paid to the issue of control, and that the external sponsors of health promotion fail to recognize the amount of power that they exert on the community. This power exists by virtue of the fact that health professionals specify – and, in some cases, supply – the goals, target groups, timescales, resources, and the organizing and accountability structures of the community development programmes. Tones and Tilford (2001) identify with this problem, referring to 'facipulation', whereby the community agenda is manipulated to effect influence on the community action. In this instance, the facilitation of an empowered community is essentially a means to an end. Such actions can be viewed as the antithesis of empowerment, which should be the primary outcome of community development (Rissel 1994; Laverack 2007). While community empowerment is clearly a desirable outcome of health promotion, its eventual aim is health improvement for the community through collective social action and political reform (Whitehead, 2004).

Health promotion as collective social action

Mittlemark (1999) asserts that an empowered community is one that has the capability to mount and manage action to improve the basic foundations for a thriving community and, often, to reduce inequity and inequality. Essentially, this embodies the intention to bring about social and political change (Laverack 2007). In doing so, collective action positively influences a community's social determinants of health (Tones and Tilford 2001). For example, Mittlemark (1999) suggests that the community might focus on equal access to education, economic security, social connectedness and the development of public policy that supports agreed objectives. Therefore, according to Whitehead (2004), health promotion is a radical socio-political process that involves activities that reinforce community action and build healthy public policy to strengthen social cohesion and social capital. These are the social components that enable belonging and trust, and can lead to improved economic performance and better health in society overall.

As Ritchie et al. (2004) point out, it is commonly agreed that appropriate leadership and effective organizational structures are crucial to successful community participation. The challenge for health promoters is to recognize the criticality of community members in the process, and to use and increase the capabilities and resources within the community. Furthermore, if they are to afford effective action, health promoters must recognize that health agendas arise from 'grass roots'. However, it would be naïve to assume that such recognition alone will lead to effective social action. Evidently, such recognition also requires a political climate that nurtures and facilitates the social-action approach, and facilitates access to education programmes, research, training and necessary resources (Ritchie et al. 2004). Furthermore, it is important to recognize that, within a community, conflicts of interest (real or imagined) might exist between disempowered people. This means that they can potentially divert the energies of disadvantaged groups into self-defeating and mutually disempowering activity. These conflicts of interest frequently require mediation by an impartial individual or group in order to facilitate empowerment.

Health promotion in action

Heenan (2004) uses evidence from a community health project that highlights the benefits and difficulties with a community development approach that aimed to facilitate community action. The community development project, based in Northern Ireland, aimed to put health on the agenda for the community and adhered to key principles of community involvement, empowerment, training, project ownership and partnership working. Heenan (2004] suggests that partnerships can positively influence a community's health status but, in order to be effective, they require considered planning and long-term commitment from both the state (political and fiscal resources) and the local community.

Making health promotion effective

The radical interpretation of health promotion is based on the assumption of the existence of power deficits or social problems in need of attention, and that these have an adverse effect on health (Bracht et al. 1999). Empowered communities have a greater impact on community health than health related work with individuals or small groups (Whitehead 2004). Together, with the commitment of professionals and communities to engage in activities, the success of 'radical' health promotion depends on the understanding that collective, rather than individual, action is needed, together with an appreciation of the relationships between power and empowerment (Tones and Tilford 2001). Health promotion is a dynamic process in which there is an acknowledgement of the necessity for collaboration and multi-agency involvement. If health promotion is to be successful, the issues of concern should be identified by the community. Therefore, there is ownership of the project by the community and active involvement of consumers at all stages. By definition, community development is linked with community, and the pre-existence of a community is clearly crucial to the success of health promotion. The capacity and capability of the community to engage in effective collective action is also a pre-requisite of radical health promotion, as this will enhance citizen participation in groups, and facilitate organizational and social action (Bracht et al. 1999).

 Tutorial brief 1.5

Think of a health promotion activity that nurses might contribute to. Identify what will need to be put in place before embarking on such an initiative.

Consequences of health promotion

The consequences of progressive health promotion are a raised level of community empowerment and the participation of empowered community members in collective political action. The attainment of outcomes that are usually sought by the community groups clusters around the desired achievement of necessary redistribution of resources, or decision-making and changes in policy to generate positive influence on social determinants of health which, ultimately, bring about the improved health of the community (Bracht et al. 1999).

Summary point

Health promotion can be viewed as a process and an outcome. The process of health promotion involves all actions that enable people to take control over their lives and their health. Progressive health promotion involves engaging in community development, either through a community-based approach that focuses on lifestyle or illness issues, or through 'true' community development where the agenda is set and the desired outcomes are identified by the community. The focus of activities is on the socio-political determinants of health and the intention is to counter the power deficits or unattended social problems that exist. The consequences of health promotion are community empowerment and participation in activities that bring about socio-political changes that positively affect the community's health.

Public health

While it is relatively straightforward to tease out the relationship between health education and health promotion through their identifying attributes, the same cannot be said for public health and health promotion. Tones and Tilford (2001) attest to the confusion by highlighting two conflicting positions: public health comprises both health promotion and public health medicine; and health promotion is the envelope that incorporates public health and public health medicine. In some respects this uncertainty might be deliberate, as there is an acknowledged – and, as yet, unresolved – power struggle between public health and health promotion (Scott-Samuel and Springett 2007). Webster and French (2002) believe this power struggle results in 'conspiratorial confusion' as health promotion specialists and public health specialists strive to protect their 'territory'. The continuing debate about the relationship between health promotion and public health could be viewed as an unnecessary preoccupation with semantics. However, the concern of a number of authors is that, rather than merely being an issue of terminology, the struggle represents intense differences over purpose and scope. The wholesale takeover of health promotion by public health – which Wills (2008) argues is the case in a number of countries – will lead to a model that moves away from the guiding values of the *Ottawa Charter* (participation, enablement and empowerment, equity and social justice) to a position that privileges epidemiology, health protection and health services improvement (Wills 2008).

It might be that nursing offers a solution to the disquiet between health promotion and public health. In 2004, in the UK, the Nursing and Midwifery Council (NMC) (the regulatory body for nursing, midwifery and health visiting) opened a three-part professional register, the Part 3 of which relates to 'specialist community public health nursing' (SCPHN). The NMC (2008) state that SCPHN's not only work with individuals and families, they also direct their work at the population level. Here, they are involved in health promotion, working in partnership and making decisions that influence the whole population. SCPHNs are engaging in community level work through projects such as 'Sure Start', an initiative established to tackle disadvantage and inequity (DfEE 1999). One of Sure Start's four main objectives is to strengthen families and communities, and it gives SCPHNs licence to work in proactive and innovative ways. The establishment of Part 3 of the NMC's register is a promising development for nurses, offering scope for work that transcends the health promotion/public health divide and enables nurses to take a legitimate role in collective social action. However, there is a danger that health promotion and public health nursing are seen solely as the business of the SCPHN, and that nurses working in other health care settings might, by default, be withdrawn from their health promotion work (see Chapter 5 for settings-based health promotion). The challenge for nursing, then, is to celebrate the success of SCPHNs as they bridge the divide between health promotion and public health, and be guided by their successes to develop health promotion initiatives in other areas of nursing.

Applying the concepts: the challenges for nurses

Health promotion researchers and practitioners recognize that the rhetoric of what is viewed as 'radical' health promotion does not always correspond with the reality of practice. Despite the fact that social, economic and environmental factors have the greatest impact on individual health, nurses' involvement in the structural level of health promotion is limited (Whitehead 2006). Because nurses' work is often tied up in dealing with ill health, they are inclined to focus on individually orientated health education activities that tend to be more compatible with 'traditional' nursing practice. This position is supported by findings from various studies that consider nurses' understanding and experiences of health promotion. For example, in the UK, Irvine (2005) and Casey (2007) both found that nurses generally impart health related information in an effort to influence the knowledge, attitudes and behaviour of their patients – thereby conforming to an individualized, health education framework. In the USA, Flocke et al. (2007) revealed a low level of utilization of team approaches and resources outside the health care setting. They concluded that a dominant acute-care approach to seeking, delivering and reimbursing health care reinforces a reactive, rather than a proactive, stance towards health promotion. Kemm (2003) points out that, in England, successive policy statements have advocated health education rather than health promotion activities, and this has probably driven nurses into a pattern of continued engagement with individual approaches. Certainly, this reported situation is not unique to any one country. However, this is not to criticize strategies that are directed at the individual, or dismiss their utility in contributing to improved health. The empowerment of individuals brings about health improvement and is a crucial step towards community empowerment. What this chapter has shown is that health education, health promotion and public health are distinct concepts, and that structural approaches lead to greater health improvement of the total population.

Conclusion

Nurses need to ensure that their health promotion interventions are based on a clear conceptual framework. The literature that has been drawn on in this chapter demonstrates that, although it is hard to pin the concepts down and produce authoritative definitions of each, it is possible to mark out boundaries that distinguish between health education, health promotion and public health. This chapter establishes the fact that nurses and other health professionals are engaged in a wealth of activities that seek to improve the health of individuals and communities. Also, depending on their process and outcome, these activities can be classified as health education, health promotion or public health. The next chapter explores health education and health promotion further by considering the theories and models that can be used to guide effective health care practice.

Additional resources

Laverack, G. and Labonte, R. (2000) 'A Planning Framework for Community Empowerment Goals within Health Promotion', *Health Policy and Planning* 15(3): 255–62.
Nutbeam, D. (1998) 'Health Promotion Glossary', *Health Promotion International*, 13(4): 349–64.
WHO (2009) Health Promotion. Available online at http://www.who.int/healthpromotion/en/ (accessed 6 March 2009).

References

Aboriginal and Torres Islander Social Justice Commissioner (2005) *Social Justice Report*, Sydney, Human Rights and Equal Opportunity Commission, cited in CSDH (2008), *Closing the Gap in a Generation: Health Equity through Action on the Social Determinants of Health*, Final Report of the Commission on Social Determinants of Health (Geneva: WHO).
BBC (2008) 'Healthy Living Can Add 14 Years'. Available online at http://news.bbc.co.uk/go/pr/fr/-/1/hi/health/7174665.stm (accessed 9 March news.bbc.co.uk/1/hi/health/7174665.stm 2009)
Bennett, P. and Murphy, S. (1997) *Psychology and Health Promotion* (Buckingham: Open University Press).
Berentson-Shaw, J. and Price, K. (2007) 'Facilitating Effective Health Promotion: Lessons from the Field', *Australian and New Zealand Journal of Public Health*, 31(1): 81–6.
Bracht, N., Kingsbury, L. and Rissel, C. (1999) 'A Five-stage Community Organisation Model for Health Promotion: Empowerment and Partnership Strategies', in Bracht, N. (ed.), *Health Promotion at the Community Level: New Advances* (Thousand Oaks, CA: Sage): 83–103.
Caraher, M. (1994) 'Nursing and Health Promotion Practice: The Creation of Victims and Winners in a Political Context', *Journal of Advanced Nursing*, 19: 465–8.
Casey, D. (2007) 'Nurses' Perceptions, Understanding and Experiences of Health Promotion', *Journal of Clinical Nursing*, 16: 1039–49.
CSDH (2008) *Closing the Gap in a Generation: Health Equity through Action on the Social Determinants of Health*, Final Report of the Commission on Social Determinants of Health (Geneva: WHO).
Dahlgren, G. and Whitehead, M. (1991) *Policies and Strategies to Promote Social Equity in Health* (Stockholm, Sweden: Institute for Future Studies).
DfEE (1999) *Making a Difference for Children and Families: Sure Start* (London: DfEE).
DHSS (1980) *Inequalities in Health: Report of a Research Group* (London: DHSS).
Dixon, J. and Sindall, C. (1994) 'Applying Logics of Challenge to the Evaluation of Community Development in Health Promotion', *Health Promotion International*, 9(4): 297–309.
Douglas, J. (2007) 'Promoting the Public Health: Continuity and Change over Two Centuries', in Douglas, J., Earle, S., Handsley, S., Lloyd, C. and Spur, S. (eds), *A Reader in Promoting Public Health: Challenge and Controversy* (Oxford :Oxford University Press): 12–18.
Earle, S. (2007) 'Promoting Public Health: Exploring the Issues', in Earle, S., Lloyd, C., Sidell, M., Spurr, S. (eds), *Theory and Research in Promoting Public Health* (London: Sage and OU Press): 1–36.

Flocke, S., Crabtree, B. and Stange, K. (2007) 'Clinician Reflections on Promotion of Healthy Behaviors in Primary Care Practice', *Health Policy*, 84: 277–83.

Georgiadis, M., Biddle, S. and Stavrou, N. (2006) 'Motivation for Weight Loss Diets: A Clustering Longitudinal Field Study using Self-esteem and Self-determination Theory Perspectives', *Health Education Journal*, 65(1): 53–72.

Gibson, C.H. (1991) 'A Concept Analysis of Empowerment', *Journal of Advanced Nursing*, 16: 354–61.

Heenan, D. (2004) 'A Partnership Approach to Health Promotion: A Case Study from Northern Ireland', *Health Promotion International*, 19(1): 105–13.

Henderson, P. and Thomas, D. (1980) *Skills in Neighbourhood Work* (London: Allen & Unwin), cited in Tones, K. and Green, J. (2004) *Health Promotion: Planning and Strategies* (London: Sage).

Huckle, T., Conway, K., Casswell, S. and Pledger, M. (2005) 'Evaluation of a Regional Community Action Intervention in New Zealand to improve Age Checks for Young People Purchasing Alcohol', *Health Promotion International*, 20(2): 147–55.

Irvine, F. (2005) 'Exploring District Nursing Competencies in Health Promotion: The Use of the Delphi Technique', *Journal of Clinical Nursing*, 14(8): 965–75.

Irvine, F. (2007) 'Examining the Correspondence of Theoretical and Real Interpretations of Health Promotion', *Journal of Clinical Nursing*, 16: 593–602.

Jensen, B.B. (1997) 'A Case of Two Paradigms within Health Education', *Health Education Research*, 12(4): 419–28.

Kemm, J. (2003) 'Health Education: A Case for Resuscitation', *Public Health*, 117: 106–11.

Labonte, R. and Robertson, A. (1996) 'Delivering the Goods, Showing our Stuff: The Case for the Constructivist Paradigm for Health Promotion Research and Practice, *Health Education Quarterly*, 23(4): 431–47.

Laverack, G. (2005) *Public Health: Power, Empowerment and Professional Practice* (Basingstoke: Palgrave Macmillan).

Laverack, G. (2007) *Health Promotion Practice: Building Empowered Communities* (Maidenhead: Open University Press).

Lazenbatt, A., Orr, J., Bradley, M., McWhirter, L. and Chambers, M. (2000) 'Tackling Inequalities in Health and Social Well-being: Evidence of 'Good Practice' by Nurses, Midwives and Health Visitors', *International Journal of Nursing Practice*, 6: 76–88.

Macdonald, G. and Bunton, R. (2002) 'Health Promotion: Disciplinary Developments', in Bunton, R. and Macdonald, G. (eds), *Health Promotion: Disciplines, Diversity and Developments*, 2nd edn (London: Routledge): 9–28.

MacDonald, T.H. (1998) *Rethinking Health Promotion: A Global Approach* (Abingdon: Routledge).

Mackenbach, J.P. (2005) *Health Inequalities: Europe in Profile*, An independent, expert report commissioned by the UK Presidency of the EU (Rotterdam: Erasmus MC University Medical Centre), cited in CSDH (2008), *Closing the Gap in a Generation: Health Equity through Action on the Social Determinants of Health*, Final Report of the Commission on Social Determinants of Health (Geneva: WHO).

McQueen, D. (1987) *Research in Health Behaviour, Health Promotion and Public Health* (Edinburgh: Edinburgh Research Unit in Health and Behavioural Change).

Mittlemark, M. (1999) 'Health Promotion at the Community Wide Level: Lessons from Diverse Perspectives', in Bracht, N. (ed.), *Health Promotion at the Community Level: New Advances* (Thousand Oaks, CA: Sage): 3–27.

NMC (2008) 'Who can be on the SCPHN Part of the Register?'. Available online at http://www.nmc-uk.org/aArticle.aspx?ArticleID=2731 (accessed 6 March 2009).

Pelletier, J., Moisan, J., Roussel, R. and Gilbert, M. (1997) 'Heart Health Promotion: A Community Development Experiment in a Rural Area of Quebec, Canada', *Health Promotion International*, 12(4): 291–8.

Peretti-Watel, P. (2005) 'Cannabis Use, Beliefs about "Hard Drugs" and "Soft Drugs" and Ineffectiveness of Anti-drug Interventions in French High Schools', *Health Education Journal*, 64(2): 142–53.

Puska, P. (1995) 'General Discussion, Recommendations and Conclusion', in Puska, P., Tuomilehto, A., Nissinen, A. and Vartiainen E. (eds), *The North Karelia Project: 20 Years Results and Experiences* (Helsinki: National Public Health Institute): 345–56.

Rankinen, T., Zuberi, A., Chagnon, Y.C., Weisnagel, S.J., Argyropoulos, G., Walts, B., Pérusse, L., and Bouchard, C. (2006) 'The Human Obesity Gene Map: The 2005 Update', *Obesity*, 14: 529–644.

Rawson, D. (2002) 'Health Promotion Theory and its Rational Reconstruction: Lessons from the Philosophy of Science', in Bunton, R. and Macdonald, G. (2002) *Health Promotion: Disciplines, Diversity and Developments*, 2nd edn (London: Routledge): 250–70.

Reidpath, D.D., Burns, C., Garrard, J., Mahoney, M., and Townsend, M. (2002) 'An Ecological Study of the Relationship between Social and Environmental Determinants of Obesity', *Health & Place*, 8(2): 141–5.

Rissel, C. (1994) 'Empowerment: The Holy Grail of Health Promotion?', *Health Promotion International*, 9(1): 39–47.

Ritchie, D., Parry, O., Gnich, W., and Platt, S. (2004) 'Issues of Participation, Ownership and Empowerment in a Community Development Programme: Tackling Smoking in a Low Income Area in Scotland', *Health Promotion International*, 19(1): 51–9.

Scott-Samuel, A. and Springett, J. (2007) 'Hegemony or Health Promotion? Prospects for Reviving England's Lost Discipline', *Journal of the Royal Society for the Promotion of Health*, 127(5): 210–13.

Seedhouse, D. (2001) *Health: The Foundations for Achievement*, 2nd edn (Chichester: John Wiley).

Sidell, M. (2000) 'Educating and Communicating through the Mass Media', in Katz, J., Peberdy, A. and Douglas, J. (eds), *Promoting Health: Knowledge and Practice* Oxford: Oxford University Press): 180–96.

Skelton, R. (1994) 'Nursing and Empowerment: Concepts and Strategies', *Journal of Advanced Nursing*, 19: 415–23.

Smith, L. and Haddad, L. (2000) *Explaining Child Malnutrition in Developing Countries: A Cross-country Analysis*, Research Report 111 (Washington, DC: International Food Policy Research Institute, cited in CSDH (2008), *Closing the Gap in a Generation: Health Equity through Action on the Social Determinants of Health*, Final Report of the Commission on Social Determinants of Health (Geneva: WHO).

Thompson, K., Parahoo, K. and Blair, N. (2007) 'A Nurse-led Smoking Cessation Clinic Quit Rate Results and Views of Participants', *Health Education Journal*, 66(4), 307–22.

Tones, K. and Green, J. (2004) *Health Promotion: Planning and Strategies*. (London: Sage).

Tones, K. and Tilford, S. (1994) *Health Education: Effectiveness, Efficiency and Equity*, 2nd edn (London: Chapman & Hall).

Tones, K. and Tilford, S. (2001) *Health Promotion: Effectiveness, Efficiency and Equity*, 3rd edn (Cheltenham: Nelson Thornes).

Weare, K. (2002) 'The Contribution of Education to Health Promotion', in Bunton, R. and Macdonald, G. (2002) *Health Promotion: Disciplines, Diversity and Developments*, 2nd edn (London: Routledge): 250–70.

Webster, C. and French, J. (2002) 'The Cycle of Conflict: The History of the Public Health and Health Promotion Movements', in Adams, L., Amos, M. and Munro, J. (eds), *Promoting Health: Policies and Practice* (London: Sage).

Whitehead, D. (2000) 'Using Mass Media within Health-promoting Practice: A Nursing Perspective', *Journal of Advanced Nursing*, 32: 807–16.

Whitehead, D. (2004) 'Health Promotion and Health Education: Advancing the Concepts', *Journal of Advanced Nursing*, 47(3): 311–20.

Whitehead, D. (2006) 'Commentary on Irvine, F. (2005) "Exploring District Nursing Competencies in Health Promotion: The Use of the Delphi Technique"', *Journal of Clinical Nursing*, 15: 649–50.

Whitehead, D. and Russell, G. (2004) 'How Effective are Health Education Programmes: Resistance, Reactance, Rationality and Risk? Recommendations for Effective Practice', *International Journal of Nursing Studies*, 41: 163–72.

Williden, M., Taylor, R., McAuley, K., Simpson, J., Oakley, M. and Mann, J. (2006) 'The APPLE Project: An Investigation of the Barriers and Promoters of Healthy Eating and Physical Activity in New Zealand Children aged 5–12 Years', *Health Education Journal*, 65(2): 135–48.

Wills, J. (2008) 'Editorial: "Health Promotion: Still Going Strong?"', *Critical Public Health*, 18(4): 431–34.

WHO (1986) *Ottawa Charter for Health Promotion* (Ottawa: WHO).

CHAPTER 2

Health Promotion Theory, Models and Approaches

Ruth Cross

Objectives

By the end of this chapter you should be able to:

- Identify and describe different approaches to promoting health with application to practice
- Explain what is meant by the terms 'theory' and 'model' as they apply to health promotion
- Identify, describe and understand central theoretical frameworks in health promotion
- Critically apply key components of health promotion theory to their practice

---

Key terms
- Community development
- Health education
- Health promotion approaches
- Health promotion models
- Health promotion theory

Introduction

The purpose of this chapter is to give the reader an accessible overview of theory in relation to health promotion in order to provide a framework that facilitates critical examination of health promotion practice. The chapter first addresses the question of what exactly an approach, theory or model is. It then it moves on to examine each of these in greater detail, drawing on relevant frameworks from the literature to illustrate the points made.

Concepts around health and health promotion underwent significant changes in the 1980s and 1990s that resulted in the creation of several different models of health promotion (Lincoln and Nutbeam 2006). Some of these will be looked at in detail in this chapter – for example, Tannahill's Model of Health Promotion (Downie *et al.* 1996), Beattie's Model of Health Promotion (Beattie 1991), Four Paradigms of Health Promotion (Caplan and Holland 1990), Pender's Health Promotion Model (Pender 1982) and Tones' Empowerment Model of Health Promotion (Tones and Tilford 2001). It is worth bearing in mind from the outset, however, that the discipline of health promotion is still relatively young in terms of theoretical development. Interestingly, after a burst of activity during the 1980s and 1990s, there has been a relative lull in recent years.

It is not the aim of this chapter to detail the many different types of theory that health promotion draws upon but, rather, to focus specifically on health promotion theory itself. An attempt is therefore made to differentiate clearly between the 'other' types of theory that are used in health promotion (for example, models of behaviour change, models of health promotion planning, and so on – see also Chapter 4) and theory that conceptualizes health promotion itself, and what health promotion 'looks like'. In other words, how we make can sense of health promotion in a logical and coherent way.

 ## Tutorial brief 2.1

Identify and list any health promotion activities within your current nursing practice. These might include activities that would be described as health education or activities that necessarily include elements of health education, but try not to focus solely on these.

Traditionally, nurses conceive of health promotion in relatively limited terms, and research seems to show that nurses tend to talk about health education rather than health promotion when asked to define and describe what health promotion is and their health promotion practice (see Chapter 1). In addition, nurses' understanding of health education and health promotion is commonly uncertain and vague, and the two terms are often used interchangeably (Whitehead 2004; Cross 2005). This might arise from difficulties with definition rather than reflecting a lack of understanding or application. As Wills (2007) argues, conceptualizing health promotion is also problematic because there are many different perspectives on health and, consequently, many different approaches to promoting health. Indeed, with new ways of educating nurses, the situation is changing; previously dominant ideas about health promotion are being challenged – particularly in the academic nursing literature (Holt and Warne 2007; Irvine 2007; Piper 2008, 2009; Whitehead 2008).

Existing research demonstrates that health promotion presents a conceptual challenge for many in practice – and not only in nursing. However, commentators such

as Whitehead (2004) document significant changes in the more recent nursing literature in terms of how health promotion is conceived. It appears that a transition might
be taking place concerning the understanding of health promotion in the nursing
profession, with a move away from the more traditional individualistic focus associated with health education towards a more socio-political and community perspective, which is more in line with the underlying principles of health promotion. Perhaps
the degree to which understanding has developed is dependent on the context in
which 'practice' is taking place. The influence and impact of space, place and setting
on health-promoting practice is significant, and is discussed in greater detail in
Chapter 5. Where any conceptual challenge exists, it is sensible to detail the theoretical frameworks that underpin the concepts. That is the main purpose of this chapter.

What are approaches to health promotion?

There are many different ways to promote health. One of the more straightforward
ways of thinking about how health promotion takes place is to consider different
approaches to health promotion. This section looks at *approaches* to health promotion in greater detail and, in doing so, considers two broad and different frameworks – one that suggests that there are *five* different approaches to health promotion
and one that suggests that there are *three*. First, the difference between top-down
and bottom-up approaches will be examined.

Top-down versus bottom-up approaches

It could be argued that much of nursing practice – at least, historically – is based on
a top-down approach whereby the health care professional is seen as the expert (or
'giver' of knowledge) and the client/patient or recipient of care is seen as a passive
participant. Power belongs with the nurse, in this case, who is seen as being the
individual who has expert knowledge and the person with the power. Expertise and
power differentials therefore flow from the nurse 'down' to the client – hence the
term 'top-down'. The client's position is therefore one of disempowerment. Latter
(2001) has highlighted the focus of top-down approaches in nursing practice,
arguing that nursing might have a tendency to disregard the patient's perspective
and encourage a passive role. The bottom-up approach is the polar opposite of the
top-down approach. Here, the roles of those involved are reversed. The client is
seen as the expert of their situation, not the health care professional, and the power
lies with the client – hence the term 'bottom-up'. This is especially the case with
community development-based interventions. Much of health promotion perceives
itself as being 'bottom-up' in terms of its values base, although there is still an
important place for top-down approaches in promoting health.

Arguably, a better way of conceiving health promotion is to think of processes
and approaches as being more equitable. Laverack (2004) has contested the two
opposing approaches of top-down and bottom-up arguing, instead, that they create
a tension for health-promotion practice. He argues for a more parallel process

whereby the power is shared between two parties and, therefore, sits neither at the 'top' nor the 'bottom'. In this context, the two approaches do not have to be seen as mutually exclusive. Rather, the 'health promoter' and the recipient are viewed as equals in the process, neither holding more power that the other (Laverack 2004).

Health promotion in action

Arneson and Ekberg (2005) demonstrate the use of a bottom-up approach to promoting health in a work-based setting. The study evaluates an intervention designed to promote employee health where the employees (participants) set their own goals and developed their own strategies to meet their goals. The result of the intervention was that the employees themselves identified their needs and the ways to address those needs, seeking out appropriate solutions. Change took place at individual, workplace and organizational levels as the participants examined their work situation, determined problems and initiated solutions. Social support and group coherence were expressed as essential in order to transform challenging strategies into action and goal realization. The findings indicate that systematic improvements of social support and group coherence among employees ought to be facilitated by the organization as a health-promoting arena.

Different approaches to promoting health

Various authors have offered different frameworks for considering approaches to health promotion. Both Naidoo and Wills (2000) and Ewles and Simnett (2003) identify five different approaches to health promotion. More recently, Wills and Earle (2007) and Sykes (2007) talk of three broad approaches to health promotion. Approaches to health promotion describe what we do when we are promoting health, and provide a framework for considering different types of health promoting practice, activity and strategies. The aim of the health promotion activity usually determines the approach – although, sometimes, the approach might determine the aim.

Naidoo and Wills (2000) describe five different approaches to health promotion: the *medical approach*, the *behaviour-change approach*, the *educational approach*, the *empowerment approach* and the *social change approach*. Ewles and Simnett (1999) also describe five distinct approaches to health promotion practice: *medical, behaviour-change, educational, client-centred* and *societal*. Both of these sets of approaches offer useful, and very similar, simplified descriptions (taxonomies) of health promotion, and each of these approaches might be described as a 'model' of health promotion. Rawson (2002) refers to these types of 'model' as iconic models whereby both a descriptive account and an application to practice are given. Rawson (2002) also makes reference to analogic models that move beyond the description that characterizes iconic models to using more abstract concepts – what health promotion might be rather than simply what it is. Analogic models, therefore, offer an opportunity to examine the underlying principles and philosophy of health promotion, as well as demonstrating what health promotion 'looks like'. Examples of analogic models will be examined later in this chapter. Using a combination of the ideas, presented by

Ewles and Simnett (2003) and Naidoo and Wills (2000), the five approaches to health promotion are discussed in turn. Naidoo and Wills' (2000) terminology for each of the five approaches is used exclusively for ease of understanding.

Medical approach

The medical approach to promoting health focuses on the prevention of ill health and early death through medical intervention. The underlying values of this approach involve a top-down way of working where the health care professional is viewed as being the expert. In this process, the 'patient' is often a passive recipient of this expertise who is expected to comply with a prescribed medically orientated regime of treatment. The medical approach is also concerned with prevention that might take place at several levels, these being: *primary prevention*, which is concerned with preventing the onset of disease (for example, screening and immunization programmes); *secondary prevention*, which is concerned with preventing the progression of a disease (for example, anti-hyperglycaemic medication to prevent the progression of diabetes); and *tertiary prevention*, which is concerned with reducing recurrence of disease or minimizing debilitating effects such as disability (for example, rehabilitation programmes).

Education approach

The education approach is fairly straightforward. The purpose is to give information to increase knowledge so that good choices for health might be made. It assumes that, by giving information, health outcomes will be improved by changes in attitudes and, ultimately, behaviour. This approach is less top-down than the medical approach in that the individual is given freedom of choice – although it might be the health care professional that actually decides what information is needed. An educational approach has been shown to be effective with regard to certain health issues. For example, in a study by Little *et al.* (2005) an educational intervention using leaflets to increase women's knowledge about contraception had a highly significant effect on the women's knowledge and a subsequent decrease in unwanted pregnancies. All health promotion activity is likely to involve some element of education. If one thinks of the term 'health education', it stands to reason that this type of approach is part of it. This is why most agree that health education is an integral component of most health promotion activity (Tones and Tilford, 2001).

Behaviour-change approach

The purpose of the behaviour-change approach is to encourage people to adopt healthier behaviours through increasing health knowledge. Increasing knowledge necessarily involves educating people – so, a link with the educational approach can be seen. Similarly also to the medical approach, the agenda is usually set by health care professionals and, again, is usually a top-down, expert led way of working. This approach focuses on trying to make people change their behaviour in some way, and makes the assumption that an increase in knowledge will create a change in behaviour. Research studies clearly show that matters are rarely quite as simple as this. One such example is the Zambia Sexual Behaviour Survey (Central Statistical Office, Ministry of Health 2002), which examined knowledge, attitudes and behaviour in relation to HIV/AIDS and sexually transmitted infections. The majority of respondents (81 per cent) indicated a high level of knowledge about how HIV transmission could be avoided. However, only a third of men and women reported having used a condom during sex with a non-regular sexual partner. Changing behaviour is much more complex than simply giving health information and expecting that to make any difference (see Whitehead and Russell 2004). This approach often blindly assumes that individuals have the power and skills to make a difference to their lives and, therefore, their own health status. However, this is rarely the case without careful planning, resources and long-term support. The behaviour-change approach is often viewed as being more individualistic and is therefore more in keeping with health education approaches (Whitehead 2001). There is a potential to 'victim blame' when using this approach.

The approaches mentioned so far (medical, educational and behavioural) have been argued to be mostly representative of different manifestations of health education activity (Whitehead 2004, 2006; Irvine 2007). The vast majority of nurses who identify themselves as being 'health-promoting' practitioners will, most probably, adopt one or more of these activities as their main area of activity.

Empowerment approach

The empowerment approach can be viewed in direct contrast to the three approaches discussed so far. The nature of the empowerment approach is that, done well, it is a more bottom-up way of approaching health promotion. In this approach, health concerns and the health priorities of individuals and social groups are identified by people themselves rather than by health care professionals. The health promoter, therefore, becomes the facilitator rather than the expert (Naidoo and Wills, 2000). Empowerment is key to health promotion practice and is an underlying principle in ways of health-promoting working. It is the process through which people gain greater control over decisions and actions affecting their health (Tones and Green 2004). Empowerment can be at an individual level (self-empowerment) or at a wider level involving groups of people (community empowerment). The latter is more likely to involve activities that are also representative of the following approach – social change.

Social change approach

The social change approach moves the focus beyond the individual to look at the wider socio-economic and political environment, which impacts on health experience. Rather than locating change as required at individual levels, the purpose

Box 2.1   Five approaches applied to obesity

Medical: Encourage people to seek medical and surgical intervention for the treatment of obesity.

Behaviour-change: Persuade people to eat more healthily and exercise more.

Education: Provide information about the importance and benefits of maintaining a 'normal' health weight and how to go about it.

Empowerment: Being overweight is only considered to be a problem if the person identifies it as one. Where guidance is sought, the nurse assists and advocates as healthy a lifestyle as possible within the parameters of being overweight. This might bring about sensible and realistic weight education – for example, facilitating self-esteem programmes.

Social change: Influencing and implementing policies to minimize the effects of an obesogenic environment – for example, clear food labelling and transport policies that encourage pedestrian activity, such as cycling.

is to effect change at societal, political or environmental levels, moving from a micro focus to a macro focus. These will then have an impact on health promotion at an individual level. Greater detail about this type of approach is offered later in this chapter (see the section on socio-environmental approaches). The empowerment and social change approaches are generally more in line with current and conventional health promotion thinking and activity.

A more accessible way of describing the five different approaches that have been presented is to try to apply each of them to a specific issue (see Box 2.1).

Tutorial brief 2.2

Consider your own practice as a health care professional. Would you say that you use a bottom-up or top-down approach, or, as Laverack (2004) suggests, do you use a 'parallel' approach? Which of the five approaches described by Naidoo and Wills (2000) and/or Ewles and Simnett (2003) would you say that you use? List the reasons why you think you use the approach that you have identified. Does your choice of approach differ according to given situations, or according to what you are trying to achieve? Would you like to change the way that you work and use a different kind of approach? If this is the case, consider how you might do this.

The three different approaches framework

Wills (2007) and Sykes (2007) present a framework of three nursing related approaches to promoting health. The resulting framework consists of three different approaches: *bio-medical, behavioural* and *socio-environmental*. This framework draws from the five-approaches framework mentioned earlier and, consequently, differs little in its nature and scope.

Biomedical approaches

The biomedical approach is similar to the medical approach. This approach focuses more on disease than on health or well-being, and therefore negative rather than positive health status. Here, the aim is to treat, ameliorate or prevent ill health. The biomedical approach is concerned with medical or clinical intervention, and is driven by scientific medicalized evidence (Sykes 2007). Again, it espouses a top-down way of working. This approach tends to target whole populations and focus on high-risk groups. Examples of these types of health promotion activity are screening and immunization. The limitation of this approach is that the wider context of people's lives is neither usually taken into account nor dealt with in terms of the impact that social determinants of health will have on people's health – housing conditions, environment and so on. In this context, a 'healthy' person is often viewed as being someone who is free of the medical risk or condition of related illness or disability.

Behavioural approaches

Behavioural approaches are largely similar to the behaviour-change approach. These approaches acknowledge that individual behaviour affects health experience. The aim is therefore to change behaviour and encourage healthier lifestyles. The focus is typically at the individual level, and still tends to be expert led and top-down in nature and scope. Again, as with a biomedical approach, there is a lack of acknowledgement of the wider context in which health behaviour occurs and the social, political, economical and ecological factors that influence an individual's health related behaviour and status.

Health promotion in action

Shankar *et al.* (2007) provide an example of a US based Washington, DC intervention designed to change dietary behaviour through educational activities. Two hundred and twelve women took part in seven classes designed to enhance knowledge and skills in relation to nutrition. Women attending the most classes (five or more out of the total seven) showed the biggest changes in terms of improvements in diet, reducing overall total calorie consumption and the percentage of calories derived from fat.

Additional point

A limitation of many behavioural-change programmes is that they often observe and measure the affects and outcomes of short-term interventions. As with the Shankar *et al.* study, there is often no means of knowing whether any of the noted changes will be permanent or only short-lived. Longer-term follow-up and evaluation can help in overcoming this dilemma (see Chapter 4).

Socio-environmental approaches

Socio-environmental approaches work in contrast to behavioural approaches in that they take the focus away from the individual (micro) level and, instead, shift the focus to structural or political (macro) levels. The intention is to create supportive environments for health, whereby it is possible for individuals to make healthier choices and sustain healthy lifestyles. This might be achieved in several different ways, such as by influencing local health policy and legislation. The health care professional might be involved in promoting health in this way through activities such as political lobbying and advocacy, and also through notions such as agenda setting and critical consciousness-raising (Whitehead 2003).

Health promotion in action

Bensberg and Kennedy (2002), in exploring the potential for health-promoting emergency departments (EDs) in Australia, highlight the need to consider socio-environmental approaches. They recommend specific activities – such as advocacy – for legislative changes and subsequent enforcement of seat belt and bicycle helmet use in communities.

Within the *social change approach*, offered by the five-approaches framework, and the *socio-environmental approach*, there are two other approaches to promoting health that are key. They are the *community development approach* and the *settings approach*.

Community development approach

Community development approaches to health promotion necessarily take into account 'lay' definitions and concepts of health, as opposed to 'professional'. They begin 'where people are at'. Community development is a political activity based on collective experience and action (Amos 2002). It is therefore viewed as being diametrically opposed to individual approaches to health promotion (health education). These, instead, focus on personal behaviour-change as the key to promoting individual health. The underpinning focus of the community development approach, therefore, centres on issues such as powerlessness and disadvantage, and the promotion of active health consumer participation and involvement. It takes place in clients' naturally occurring environments – that is, where they live, work and play. Concurrent with a key aim of health promotion, the purpose of this approach is to address injustices and inequalities in society. Community development is, therefore, concerned with critical consciousness-raising and change. Community development is also a philosophy, as well as a way of working (Amos 2002). At first, it might not appear that this approach to promoting health has much relevance to nursing. However, authors such as Whitehead (2003) argue that it has. It might be that the perceived value of this type of approach within nursing is dependent on the context in which the nursing activity takes place. Rightly or wrongly, for instance, with those who work within community settings feeling more akin to this approach than those who work in acute settings (Cross 2005). Amos (2002: 64) argues that:

> the distinctive contribution of the community development approach ... is that the focus is on increasing equity and access which challenges medical power.

Working with communities is crucial to this approach, but there are further considerations to take into account. Community development approaches might not be a panacea for all eventualities.

While the community development approach espouses key health promotion principles, Robinson and Elliott (2000: 219) argue that evidence of their use is limited. They conducted a qualitative study in Ottawa, Canada, exploring the factors affecting the use of community development approaches to heart health. They go on to state that no single community approach is appropriate for all health promotion initiatives, and conclude that 'it may not be realistic to advocate community development as the goal to which all communities should strive'.

 Tutorial brief 2.3

Consider the community development approach. What do you think might be the advantages and disadvantages of using this approach to promote health? Make a list and consider this in relation to your own role.

Settings approach

The settings approach is another means by to accomplish health promotion. This approach considers the places and spaces where people's lives are enacted and is, therefore, essentially concerned with where health promotion takes place. The interconnection of different settings and how they impact on the health status of all people is an important consideration in health promotion. Chapter 5 is devoted to detailing the settings-based approach to health promotion.

Health promotion in action

Haines *et al.* (2006) carried out an evaluation on a multi-component intervention implemented in the school setting designed to prevent teasing and unhealthy weight control behaviour among adolescents. The intervention focused on activities promoting a 'no-teasing' message and necessarily had to take place within this setting in order to focus specifically on the target group. The outcome was a significant reduction in the number of students reporting teasing.

A combination of approaches?

In practice, quite often, a combination of approaches is used in health promotion interventions. It can sometimes be difficult to distinguish between different approaches and it is rare to see one type of approach being used exclusively. In addition, different approaches might be relevant at different times, depending on the aim of the health promotion intervention. There is no right or wrong way to carry out health promotion and all approaches have the potential to be effective in promoting health – if carefully planned, structured, implemented and evaluated (see Chapter 4). The important thing to note is that the use of a particular approach to promoting health usually reflects a particular viewpoint or set of values guiding our practice as health promoters and health educators. Health promotion is a collaborative process that cannot be practised by individual health professionals acting in isolation. It is worth noting that the case is the same for effective health education. Therefore, the adopted approach will usually accommodate the differing values and principles of a number of practitioners and the clients that they serve. Of course, the nature of the approach adopted, on the notion that 'health' itself is something that is worth promoting, is essential.

Summary point

Health promotion can take place in different ways and one way of conceptualizing this is to consider different approaches to promoting health. Approaches describe what health promoters do and a combination of approaches is often used in practice.

Health promotion theory and models

The next section of this chapter considers specific theoretical frameworks (models) in health promotion. Before several models are examined in some detail, we need to be clear about what it meant by the terms 'theory' and 'model'. The interchangeable use of these terms can commonly lead to confusion. Lucas and Lloyd (2005) point out that, in their experience, the terms 'theory', 'model', 'evidence' and 'approach' are all often used interchangeably. However, they are tolerant of this situation where it occurs, stating that 'all are attempts to guide health promotion activity by some kind of rationale'.

What is health promotion theory?

Health promotion theory serves to capture the nature of health promotion in some way and, therefore, to provide a framework for describing and analyzing what the processes, activity and content of health promotion actually are. Health promotion theory is most probably used to understand or examine health promotion practice, and to provide a framework for systematically doing so.

Tones and Green (2004) distinguish between different types of theory in health promotion: *normative theory* and *analytical theory*. Normative theory can be explained as theory that is a description of what is involved in health promotion, and thus aims to simply represent or describe reality. On the other hand, analytical theory refers to health promotion theory that goes beyond description of health promotion activity to analyzing the underlying principles of practice (Wills and Earle 2007). Understanding the theory that underpins health promotion helps us to better understand what health related activities we are engaging in, and when we are or are not conducting health promotion.

Nutbeam and Harris (2004) argue that the potential of theory to guide the development of health promotion interventions is substantial. In addition to enabling us to understand and explain what health promotion is about, Wills and Earle (2007) suggest that theory might be used for analytical, predictive and explanatory purposes. They provide a useful framework for understanding what theory is about and propose that theory is helpful in addressing questions such as 'What is it?' (description); 'Why is it?' (explanatory); 'What would happen if?' (predictive) and 'What should be done?' (prescriptive). Of course, as Tones and Green (2004) argue, we should bear in mind that this might only be the case with 'good' or 'sound' theory. Poorly conceived theory is unlikely to answer any questions or resolve issues.

What is a 'model'?

Models might evolve or derive from theory and are attempts to represent reality. Models might also be referred to as abstract conceptualizations. Think of a model railway or an architect's model of a building that try to represent the 'real' thing in some way. Models can be seen to help to understand what something looks like, even before it exists, and what its key characteristics or components are. In this case, it refers to health promotion that is under consideration – that is, what *does* health promotion look like – or even, what *could* health promotion look like?

As with theory, models can describe, explain, predict or prescribe (Wills and Earle 2007). Models can also be used to develop and assist understanding. As Sykes (2007) argues, by providing a theoretical structure with which health promotion

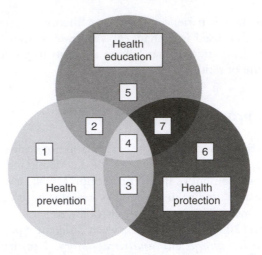

Figure 2.1 Tannahill's model of health promotion
Source: Downie et al. (1996) reproduced with the permission of Oxford University Press.

can be examined, models assist in the consideration of a range of perspectives on health – as well as the philosophy, values and beliefs that impact on health promotion practice. In addition, Sykes (2007) suggests that models of health promotion offer the potential to question practice and its underlying assumptions. However, she cautions against viewing models of health promotion practice in the same light as nursing models.

Health promotion models

As Naidoo and Wills (2005) argue, models help to perform a number of important functions. Among other things, models of health promotion can be used to examine health promotion practice and to plan interventions. The next section focuses on several specific contemporary theoretical frameworks or 'models' of health promotion.

Tannahill's model of health promotion

Tannahill's model of health promotion (Downie *et al.* 1996) is intended as a framework for defining, planning and carrying out health promotion, and has been widely used since its inception. As can be seen in Figure 2.1, health promotion comprises three overlapping domains or 'spheres' of activity – *health education*, *prevention* and *health protection*. The model distinguishes between seven different areas or domains of health promotion activity. These are:

1 Prevention – which includes activities such as screening and immunization;
2 Health education for prevention – which includes activities such as those that try to encourage the uptake of preventive measures;

3   Preventive health protection – which includes activities such as putting fluoride in water to prevent tooth decay;
4   Health education for preventive health protection – which includes activities such as discouraging smoking in indoor places through policy;
5   Health education – which includes activities aimed at changing behaviour through education; for example, providing information about the benefits of a healthy diet;
6   Health protection – which includes activities such as the provision of non-smoking workplaces;
7   Health education for health protection – which includes a policy commitment to promoting health.

In Tannahill's model, health promotion activity is identified as being one of these types (or within these 'domains') of activity or, indeed, as a combination of them. The model therefore emphasizes the wide range of activities that can be identified as 'health promotion', and also the fact that many health promotion activities 'overlap' or even complement each other. The main strength of this model is that is it relatively easy to understand and offers a clear conceptualization of what health promotion looks like. However, it is also criticized for being over-simple and descriptive, and does not offer any explanation of underlying principles or values in health promotion practice.

Beattie's model of health promotion

Beattie (1991) provides a different kind of theoretical framework for health promotion. The model specifically focuses on interventions rather than activity *per se* and is presented as four quadrants. Each quadrant comprises a different area of health promotion activity. Crucial to the model are the two axes running through the middle. The horizontal axis represents the focus of the intervention (as being on a continuum from 'individual' to 'collective') and the vertical axis represents the mode of intervention (as being on a continuum from 'negotiated' to 'authoritative'). The axes bisect to form the four quadrants.

Additional point

Note that the vertical axis can be seen to reflect the top-down (expert led) and bottom-up (participatory) approaches referred to previously in this chapter. Note also that the bottom left hand quadrant – 'Community Development' – has similarities to the community development approach discussed earlier.

Beattie terms the quadrants *health persuasion, personal counselling, legislative action* and *community development* respectively (see Figure 2.2). Legislative action and

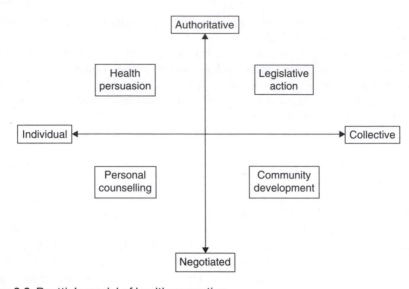

Figure 2.2 Beattie's model of health promotion
Source: Beattie (1991) reproduced with the permission of Taylor & Francis Books UK.

community development are deemed to be more collective types of health promotion and sit on the right-hand side of the model. Legislative action relates more to the political and health policy arm of community development, and this is indicated by its positioning in the model. Legislative action refers to interventions that aim to enable healthier choices or, in fact, sometimes take away choice in the name of health improvement. Recent bans on smoking in indoor public places in many countries are a good example of how choice has been restricted to improve health. Community development refers to activity or interventions that involve communities themselves and that aim to empower groups to effect change through addressing issues such as inequity and inequality.

Personal counselling and health persuasion sit on the left-hand side of the model, and reflect activity or interventions aimed more at the individual (health education) level. Personal counselling is concerned with empowerment at the individual level, and the impression of negotiation is given here. Sykes (2007) suggests that nurses have traditionally been associated with fairly authoritarian, top-down interventions. However, others such as Scriven (2005) and Whitehead (2005) argue that nurses have the potential to be far more involved in participatory activities – such as with action research (see Chapters 4 and 6). In terms of the focus of the interventions in Beattie's model, it could be argued that nurses' health promotion activity tends traditionally to focus on the individual. Thus, much of health promotion from nurses' perspectives is said to be located on the left-hand side of the vertical axis and mainly within the 'health persuasion' quadrant of the model.

An important thing to note about Beattie's (1991) model is that it locates health promotion within the wider social, political and cultural context in which it takes place, and suggests that health promotion cannot be removed from this. Beattie

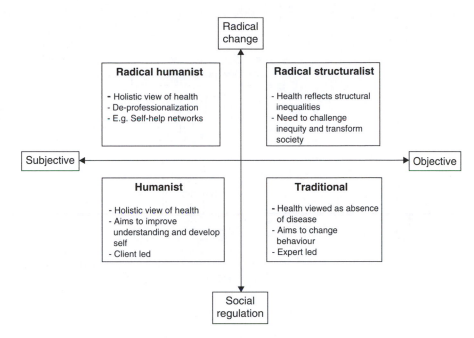

Figure 2.3 Four paradigms of health promotion
Source: Adapted from Caplan and Holland (1990) reproduced with the permission of Sage Publications Ltd.

actually locates each quadrant of activity in the political arena by giving each one a different label in terms of ideology. This clearly reflects the political nature of health promotion, and is a useful way to consider principles and values within health promotion practice. However, all health promotion activity, reflected by the four quadrants, is essentially concerned with trying to change or control behaviour in some way – albeit employing different means to do so.

Caplan and Holland's four paradigms of health promotion

Caplan and Holland (1990) offer a more detailed political view of health promotion in their model. Similar to Beattie's (1991) model, Caplan and Holland offer a framework of health promotion comprising four quadrants bisected by two axes. The vertical axis represents the *nature of society* – or, what society is like, and whether there is conflict or consensus. The horizontal axis represents the *nature of knowledge* – or, ways of knowing, and whether these are subjective or objective. Mapping the axes onto each other results in four quadrants each representing a different perspective. These four quadrants are called *radical humanist, radical structuralist, humanist* and *traditional* (see Figure 2.3). Interestingly, Wills and Earle (2007) note that the four quadrants representing different forms of health promotion are similar to Ewles and Simnett's five approaches.

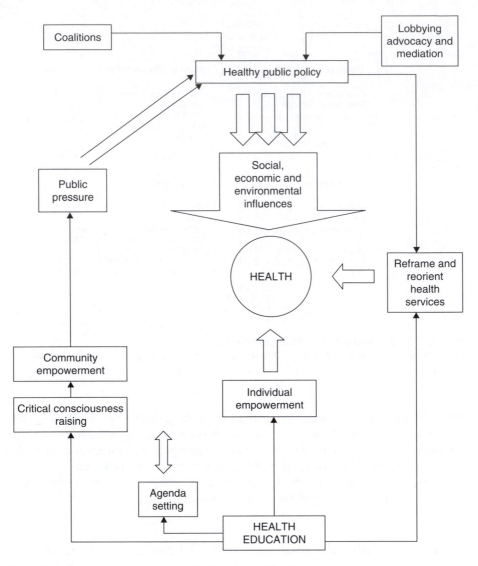

Figure 2.4 An empowerment model of health promotion
Source: Tones and Tilford (2001) reproduced with the permission of Nelson Thornes Ltd.

Tones' empowerment model of health promotion

The empowerment model of health promotion, as conceptualized by Tones and Tilford (see Figure 2.4), is built around the relationship between health education and healthy public policy. Thus, health promotion is a combination of health education and healthy public policy. These are the key concepts demonstrated in their often quoted equation: 'Health Promotion = Health Education x Healthy Public Policy'. The model is based on the *health field concept*, introduced by the then Canadian Health Minister Marc Lalonde in the 1970s, and takes into account four key influences on health: *genetic influences, environmental influences, lifestyle influences* and *influences of medical services* (Lalonde 1974). Policy is seen as key in addressing socio-economic, environmental and cultural factors influencing health, as well as impacting on health service quality and delivery. The model includes two other key areas: political lobbying and advocacy, and political mediation. Central to the model is the notion of social empowerment and enabling people to gain control over their health, with the main premise being to increase the autonomy of the individual. The model is more in line with community empowerment and social approaches to health promotion, rather than with trying to use persuasive measures to change behaviour.

Pender's Health Promotion Model

Pender's Health Promotion Model (HPM) (Pender 1982) (see Figure 2.5) is described as a competence (or approach oriented model), and brings together a nursing and behavioural science perspective on factors influencing health behaviours (Pender *et al.* 2006). It is the only nursing-specific model that has been described so far. The model draws heavily on expectancy value theory, similar to the well-known Health Belief Model (Becker 1974) (based on socio cognitive theory), and incorporates concepts from these frameworks within a nursing perspective of holistic human functioning.

The model includes seven cognitive-perceptual factors and five modifying factors that are used to explain and predict health behaviours (see Box 2.2).

Many of the variables within the HPM have been used in nursing research into health behaviour. The model was later revised to include three new variables: *activity-related effect, commitment to a plan of action* and *immediate competing demands and preferences*. While this model is called a model of health promotion, it might actually sit more comfortably within models or theories of behaviour-change – albeit more explanatory and analytical than descriptive (see earlier discussion and Chapter 4). However, it is acknowledged that health-promoting behaviour is the endpoint or action outcome of the HPM (Pender *et al.* 2006). It should be noted that this model was developed with a specific health care system in mind and, therefore, is contextual. This might provide an explanation for its stronger alliance and allegiance with a more health education oriented perspective.

Additional point

Pender's Health Promotion Model might actually be more accurately described as a model of behavioural change – in other words, a Health Education Model.

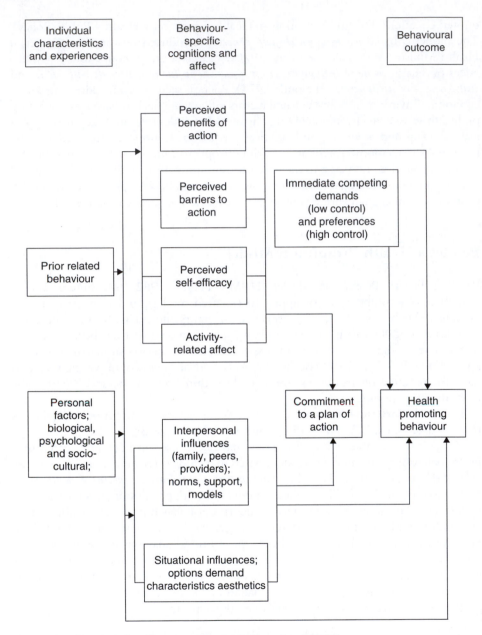

Figure 2.5 Pender's health promotion model – revised (2006)
Source: Pender et al. (2006) reproduced with the permission of Pearson Education, Inc.

Box 2.2   Factors in Pender's Health Promotion Model

Cognitive-perceptual factors:

- The importance of health
- Perceived control of health
- Definition of health
- Perceived health status
- Perceived self-efficacy
- Perceived benefits
- Perceived barriers

Modifying factors:

- Demographic characteristics
- Biological characteristics
- Interpersonal influences
- Situational influences
- Behavioural factors

Tutorial brief 2.4

Consider your health promotion practice in relation to one of the theories of health promotion that have been outlined. Where does your practice fit? For example, if you choose to examine your practice using Beattie's model, which quadrant does it fall into? What are the advantages of working in this way? What are the possible limitations? Make a list of each. Would you like to work in different ways? Consider the reasons why? How might you achieve this?

Summary point

Different models of health promotion exist within the literature. Care should be taken to distinguish between models of health education and models of health promotion, as these are not necessarily the same thing.

Several different models of health promotion have been considered in this chapter. They are not exhaustive but they are among the more contemporary models in the literature. There are, subsequently, other models that you might come across in the wider health promotion literature that are not covered in this chapter. In addition, a wide variety of different theory underpins health promotion practice and informs the development, implementation and evaluation of health promotion interventions. Health promotion theory draws on theory from other disciplines – such as psychology, sociology, social policy and communication, to name but a few. Nutbeam and Harris (2004) offer a succinct overview of the range of health promotion theory used in practice. The range of health promotion theory, using Nutbeam and Harris's (2004) guide, includes theories on health behaviour and health behaviour change, theories on change in communities and communal action for health, theories for communication to bring about behaviour change, theories for change in organization and for the creation of health-supportive organization practice and, finally, theories for the development of healthy public policy.

Additional point

In relation to health promotion theory and models of health promotion itself – or what health promotion looks like – it is interesting to note that there has been an apparent lack of theoretical advances since the 1990s. There is still scope for the development of further theoretical frameworks and theory in examining health promotion – especially in the health service professions.

 ### Tutorial brief 2.5

Drawing on the contents of this chapter, and the work you have done in the previous tutorial briefs, identify the key elements that comprise your own health promotion practice. Can you devise a model or theoretical framework that illustrates this? Is your model mainly descriptive, explanatory, predictive or prescriptive? To what extent does it do each of these things?

Summary point

While the terms 'theory' and 'models' are often used interchangeably, it is possible to distinguish, to some extent, between the two concepts. Theory can comprise a set of concepts, principles and constructs, while models provide a framework or structure by which the relationships between different theoretical aspects are presented.

Conclusion

This chapter started off by considering different approaches to promoting health and progressed to focusing specifically on health promotion theories and models. It has examined different frameworks that are used within the literature that describe and explain what health promotion is and how it might work. What is focused on here are the theoretical frameworks (models) of health promotion rather than the range of other theory that health promotion draws on from related disciplines such as psychology, sociology, social policy, epidemiology and change-communication. The underlying values and principles of health promotion have also been discussed, where appropriate, in terms of understanding different concepts and the basis for different models.

Additional resource

Davies, M. and Macdowall, W. (2006) *Health Promotion Theory* (Maidenhead: Open University Press).

References

Amos, M. (2002) 'Community Development', in Adams, L., Amos, M. and Munro, J. (eds), *Promoting Health: Politics and Practice* (London: Sage): 63–71.
Arneson, H. and Ekberg, K. (2005) 'Evaluation of Empowerment Processes in a Workplace Health Promotion Intervention based on Learning in Sweden', *Health Promotion International*, 20: 351–9.
Beattie, A. (1991) 'Knowledge and Control in Health Promotion: A Test Case for Social Policy and Social Theory', in Gaber, J., Calnam, M., Bury, M. (eds), *The Sociology of the Health Service* (London: Routledge).
Becker, M.H. (1974) *The Health Belief Model and Personal Health Behaviour* (Thorofare, NJ: Charles B. Slack).
Bensberg, M. and Kennedy, M. (2002) 'A Framework for Health Promoting Emergency Departments', *Health Promotion International*, 17: 172–88.
Caplan, R. and Holland, R. (1990) 'Rethinking Health Education Theory', *Health Education Journal*, 49(1), 10–12.
Central Statistical Office, Ministry of Health (2002) *Zambia Sexual Behaviour Survey 2000*, April (Place: USAID).
Cross, R. (2005) 'Accident and Emergency Nurses' Attitudes to Health Promotion', *Journal of Advanced Nursing*, 51: 474–83.
Downie, R.S., Tannahill, C. and Tannahill, A. (1996) 'Health Promotion, Models and Values', 2nd edn (Oxford: Oxford University Press).
Ewles, L. and Simnett, I. (1999) *Promoting Health: A Practical Guide*, 4th edn (London: Ballière Tindall).
Ewles, L. and Simnett, I. (2003) *Promoting Health: A Practical Guide*, 5th edn (London: Ballière Tindall).
Haines, J., Neumark-Sztainer, D. and Cheryl, L. (2006) 'V.I.K. (Very Important Kids): A School-based Programme designed to Reduce Teasing and Unhealthy Weight-control Behaviours', *Health Education Research*, 21: 884–95.
Holt, M. and Warne, T. (2007) 'The Educational and Practice Tensions in Preparing Pre-registration Nurses to become Future Health Promoters: A Small-scale Explorative Study', *Nurse Education in Practice*, 7: 373–80.
Irvine, F. (2007) 'Examining the Correspondence of Theoretical and Real Interpretations of Health Promotion', *Journal of Clinical Nursing*, 16(3): 593–602.
Lalonde, M. (1974) *A New Perspective on the Health of Canadians* (Ottowa: Ministry of National Health and Welfare).
Latter, S. (2001) 'The Potential for Health Promotion in Hospital Nursing Practice', in Scriven, A. and Orme, J. (eds), *Health Promotion: Professional Perspectives* (Basingstoke: Palgrave Macmillan).

Laverack, G. (2004) *Health Promotion Practice: Power and Empowerment* (London: Sage).

Lincoln, P. and Nutbeam, D. (2006) 'WHO and International Initiatives', in Davies, M. and Macdowall, W. (eds) (2006) *Health Promotion Theory* (Maidenhead: Open University Press): 16–23.

Little, P., Griffin, S., Kelly, J., Dickson, N. and Sadler. C. (2005) 'Effect of Educational Leaflets and Questions on Knowledge of Contraception in Women taking the Combined Contraceptive Pill: Randomised Controlled Trial', *BMJ*, 316: 1948–52.

Lucas, K. and Lloyd, B. (2005) *Health Promotion: Evidence and Experience* (London: Sage).

Naidoo, J. and Wills, J. (2000) *Health Promotion: Foundations for Practice*, 2nd edn (London: Baillière Tindall).

Naidoo, J. and Wills, J. (2005) *Public Health and Health Promotion: Developing Practice*, 2nd edn (London: Baillière Tindall).

Nutbeam, D. and Harris, E. (2004) *Theory in a Nutshell: A Practical Guide to Health Promotion theories*, 2nd edn (London: McGraw-Hill).

Pender, N.J. (1982) *Health Promotion in Nursing Practice* (Norwalk, CT: Appleton-Century-Crofts).

Pender, N.J., Murdaugh, C.L. and Parsons, M.A. (2006) *Health Promotion in Nursing Practice*, 5th edn (New Jersey: Pearson Prentice Hall).

Piper, S. (2008) 'A Qualitative Study Exploring the Relationship between Nursing and Health Promotion Language, Theory and Practice', *Nurse Education Today*, 28: 186–93.

Piper, S. (2009) *Health Promotion for Nurses: Theory and Practice* (Abingdon: Routledge).

Rawson, D. (2002) 'Health Promotion Theory and its Rational Construction: Lessons from the Philosophy of Science', in Bunton, R. and Macdonald, G. (eds), *Health Promotion: Disciplines, Diversity and Developments*, 2nd edn (London: Routledge).

Robinson, K.L. and Elliott, S.J. (2000) 'The Practice of Community Development Approaches in Heart Health Promotion', *Health Education Research*, 15: 219–31.

Scriven, A. (2005) 'Promoting Health: A Global Context and Rationale', in Scriven, A. and Garman, S. (eds), *Promoting Health: Global Perspectives* (London: Palgrave MacMillan): 1–13.

Shankar, S., Klassen, A.C., Garrett-Mayer, E., Houts, P.S., Wang, T., McCarthy, M., Cain, R. and Zhang, L. (2007) 'Evaluation of a Nutrition Education Intervention for Women Residents of Washington, DC, Public Housing Communities', *Health Education Research*, 22: 425–37.

Sykes, S. (2007) 'Approaches to Promoting Health', in Wills, J. (ed.) *Promoting Health. Vital Notes for Nurses* (Oxford: Blackwell).

Tones, K. and Green, J. (2004) *Health Promotion: Planning and Strategies* (London: Sage).

Tones, K. and Tilford, S. (2001) *Health Promotion: Effectiveness, Efficiency and Equity*, 3rd edn (Cheltenham: Nelson Thornes).

Whitehead, D. (2001) 'A Socio-cognitive Approach for Health Education/Health Promotion Practice', *Journal of Advanced Nursing*, 36: 417–25.

Whitehead, D. (2003) 'Incorporating Socio-political Health Promotion Activities in Nursing Practice', *Journal of Clinical Nursing*, 12: 668–77.

Whitehead, D. (2004) 'Health Promotion and Health Education: Advancing the Concepts', *Journal of Advanced Nursing*, 47: 311–20.

Whitehead, D. (2005) 'The Culture, Context and Progress of Health Promotion in Nursing', in Scriven, A. (ed.), *Health Promoting Practice: The Contribution of Nurses and Allied Health Professionals* (Basingstoke: Palgrave Macmillan).

Whitehead, D. (2006) 'Health Promotion in the Practice Setting: Findings from a Review of Clinical Issues', *Worldviews on Evidence-based Nursing*, 3: 165–84.

Whitehead, D. (2008) 'An International Delphi Study examining Health Promotion and Health Education in Nursing Practice, Education and Policy', *Journal of Clinical Nursing*, 17: 891–900.

Whitehead, D. and Russell, G. (2004) 'How Effective are Health Education Programmes – Resistance, Reaction, Rationality and Risk? Recommendations for Effective Practice', *International Journal of Nursing Studies*, 41: 163–72.

Wills, J. (2007) 'Introduction: The Role of the Nurse in Promoting Health', in Wills, J. (ed.), *Promoting Health. Vital Notes for Nurses*. (Oxford: Blackwell).

Wills, J. and Earle, S. (2007) 'Theoretical Perspectives on Promoting Public Health', in Earle, S., Lloyd, C.E., Sidell, M. and Spurr, S. (eds), *Theory and Research in Promoting Public Health* (Milton Keynes: Open University).

CHAPTER 3

Health Promotion and the Role and Function of the Nurse

Tony Warne and Sue McAndrew

Objectives

By the end of this chapter you should be able to:

- Understand the professional and political context for nurses adopting health-promoting approaches to practice
- Recognize the organizational, educational and personal factors that might inhibit or increase effectiveness as a health-promoting nurse
- Understand the scope for change in an individual's sense of health and well-being through effective nursing care and health-promoting practice

---

Key terms
- Action-learning
- Health-promoting nursing practice
- Health promotion – nursing role and function
- Health promotion – understanding and doing
- Organizational, professional and personal barriers to health promotion
- Role models
- Self-awareness

Introduction

It was Florence Nightingale who said that she looked forward to a time when nurses would not only be there for the sick, but for also for the well. This bold idea is as important today as it was back in 1892. Just over a century after Florence Nightingale made her observation, the World Health Organization (WHO 2000) called for health promotion to be an explicit feature of pre-registration nurse training and education. Unfortunately, nurses are not always good role models in terms of health promotion and illness-prevention behaviours. For example, in two studies exploring attitudes of nurses towards smoking, a significant number of nurses did not appreciate that effective role modelling involved not smoking, and promoting a non-smoking lifestyle (Clark et al. 2003; McCann et al. 2005). Interestingly, despite there being a strong link between a healthy nursing workforce and improved patient health (O'Brien-Pallas and Baumann, 2000; Whitehead 2006), many of the organizations nurses work in do not actively try to promote the health and well-being of individual nurses (Watson 2006). Perhaps, then, there are other reasons why nurses have not seized Florence Nightingale's vision.

This chapter aims to explore what some of these reasons might be. It starts by giving a context for health promotion and health education in relation to nursing, and considers what opportunities there might be for nurses to use a health promotion approach in their everyday practice. Finally, the chapter explores some of the practical responses that would enable all nurses to be more pro-active in using health-promoting approaches as an integral part of their everyday practice. Intentionally, an important focus of this chapter, as it is an issue that is often ignored by other health promotion texts, is related to the context of *self* and attitudes around personal health. We need to know our health-promoting selves before we can influence the health-promoting ways of others.

Who does health promotion?

The idea that nurses are in a prime position to contribute to the health improvement of individuals and communities has been a consistent feature of international health care policy. Scriven and Garman (2005) have explored the global developments in health promotion policy and practice. They note that, over the past thirty years, there has been a growing emphasis on public health and health promotion in these policies. There are three strands to be found in these policies:

1. When health care is required, it will be provided by the state or government.
2. Health care will be evidence based and universally provided against agreed standards.
3. Equally, investment and attention needs to be paid to illness-preventing initiatives.

Point 3 extends the traditional understanding of what many nurses understand their practice to be concerned with, moving them into the realms of health promotion (Jordan 2000). These policies have also significantly influenced the educational curricula of pre- and post-registration nursing programmes, placing greater emphasis on health promotion and the prevention of ill health as an activity that is integral to all health care professional practice. Similarly, other guidelines, (DoH 2004; RCN 2007) suggest the direction and expansion of public health nursing in practice as being the focus of interest in primary and community based nursing teams, in collaboration with the wider primary health care team. While public health concerns itself with the prevention and eradication of disease and the wider socio-cultural context in which it occurs (see Chapter 1), most nurses (most of whom are still hospital based) confine themselves to the domains of health promotion and health education that align closely with their everyday practice (Borchardt 2000).

As outlined in Chapter 1, health promotion can be viewed as an 'umbrella term' that has often been used interchangeably with concepts of health education and illness prevention. Traditionally, in many countries, health promotion and health education have largely been associated with nursing groups such as public health nurses, practice nurses, health visitors and school nurses (Holt and Warne 2007). However, in keeping with global trends, current Western policy guidance (DoH 2004; 2006) points to the need for a new vision for nurse led health promotion, advice and education within all primary, secondary and tertiary care settings. It could be argued that the achievement of these policy ideals will require some radical changes to pre- and post-registration curricula and the way in which clinical placement experiences are supported (Jordan 2000). It has been suggested that traditional professional training, undertaken by many health service staff, often falls short of including an overt focus on health improvement or highlighting opportunities for staff to engage patients in improving their health (DoH 2004). The curriculum should be a significant building block for enhancing pre-registration nurses' knowledge about health promotion and health education within a framework of public health, thus providing the foundation for continuous professional development and life-long learning (Carr 2008; Piper 2008). Current pre-registration nursing programmes are quite varied in their health education and health promotion content (Latter and Westwood 2001; Carr 2008). Studies have shown that, despite the inclusion of health promotion theory in its broadest sense within pre-registration curricula, many nurses continue to conceptualize health promotion in relation to behaviour-change and lifestyle practices (Macleod-Clarke and Maben, 1998; Holt and Warn, 2007). This narrower view of health promotion adds further to the confusion and, for some nurses, causes ambiguity in identifying what role they should adopt with regard to this aspect of their work (Norton, 1998) (see Chapter 1).

Shifting the nurse's knowledge and understanding of health promotion

Health promotion, historically an integral component of nursing practice, has evolved in tandem with recent conceptual innovations in health care resulting from a shift in emphasis on disease toward one of wellness (Rush 2002). The traditional preventive model, largely medically driven, was concerned with preventing disease by presenting people with information about the risks of certain behaviours and lifestyle choices on their health. Here, the focus is primarily on individuals taking greater responsibility for their own health. Indeed, recent policy guidance in the UK, such as that contained in *Our Health, Our Care, Our Say* (DoH 2006), implicitly and explicitly shifted responsibility onto individual citizens to take greater responsibility for their own health and lifestyle choices. The consequences of not doing so were presented as the spectre of scarcity, with health care resources not being available to the individual as and when they might be required. For example, those who are obese might be precluded from certain operations. Nurses have both to receive these types of messages and to learn to adjust their practice in response to this policy shift (Rutherford et al. 2005). Thus, whereas traditional illness based health promotion approaches were mainly those concerned with health education, contemporary professional nursing practice has subsequently expanded to include those roles of consultant, advocate, mediator, case manager, supporter, partner and social activist – in response to these policy shifts (ICN 2000). These responses are reminiscent of the move towards an approach to health education and health promotion that can be described as critical consciousness-raising. Here, the emphasis, in terms of health-promoting activities, is located in supportive, empowering and non-judgemental relationships. In using such an approach, health education becomes part of health promotion and its effectiveness at an individual and community level, and is enhanced by a supportive policy agenda (Carr 2008). Nurses are becoming more and more aware of these positions, and are becoming either more visible in these roles or are preparing to springboard themselves into them.

Given a supportive policy context, nurses now have the opportunity to revisit their previous health-promoting role in order to avoid simplistic and tokenistic improvements (Warne et al. 2006). Nurses are now also more involved in creating greater awareness of how health might be determined and experienced, promoting caring organizational environments that provide and foster support, helping individuals to develop personal skills that enhance their ability to consider healthier choices, and building relationships with other health and social care professionals that can more effectively promote health and well-being across whole communities. Thus, nurses are beginning to think beyond health promotion work that is only carried out within specialist services, or is confined to specific responses to disease and illness, so as to adopt a more widespread and holistic approach (Holt and Warne 2007; Olshansky 2007). The next section in the chapter explores a number of organizational, professional and personal factors that might impact on a nurse's response to the policy drivers for developing health-promoting nursing practice.

 Tutorial brief 3.1

Think about a patient you have nursed who, on reflection, might have benefited from a health-promoting activity. From your personal perspective, write down all the things that might have prevented you from engaging in this activity with the patient at that time. Now, devise a table that has three columns: organizational, professional and personal. Try to put each of the things that prevented you from engaging in health promotion activity under each heading. Reflect on the possible relationships between the factors set out in each of the columns and how they would impact on your practice. For example, some nurses have more autonomy over what they do while at work; this can often allow the individual more control over prioritizing their time and interactions with patients. Which of these columns do you think it would be easiest for you to change in the future?

Organizational, professional and personal barriers to developing health-promoting practice

Where an individual spends their working day can impact upon their sense of well-being, and promote or inhibit their physical and mental health. There are a number of physical and psychological factors that contribute to the individual's reaction to their working environment (Carlson and Warne 2007). In the context of nursing, the evidence suggests a connection between the working environment and nurses' health or ill health and perceived level of well-being (Wright 2000; Baumann et al. 2001; Shamian 2005) (see Chapter 5 for more detail on workplace health promotion). Workplaces, such as the hospital and other health and social care settings, are often experienced by nurses as 'harmful'. Health care settings can be physically and mentally demanding because of long hours, heavy workloads, staffing problems, insufficient resources, low pay, lack of respect, exclusion from decision-making, and conflict (Baumann et al. 2001; Carlson and Warne 2007). For many individuals, there can be the emotional burden of working with individuals who are experiencing pain, physical and/or emotional, anxiety, and loss – which often goes unnoticed or is assumed to be part of the emotional labour of health work (Warne and McAndrew 2008). Coping with this burden can affect the quality of nurse patient relationships, job satisfaction and can even result in illness on the part of the nurse (Wright 2000; Warne and McAndrew 2007, 2008).

A number of areas of concern have been noted in the literature as barriers to working in a health-promoting way. These can be: 'horizontal violence' (activities such as defensiveness, not being allowed to carry out the activities considered the work of others, in-fighting and bullying) (Stokols et al. 1996); the internalization of societal values over the altruistic nature of nurses' work, demonstrated as denial of the worth of caring ('a virtuous silence') (Buresh and Gordon 2000: 32), and self-effacing behaviours such as 'making do' with inadequate resources – including time, money, and people (Rutherford et al. 2005). In all of these disempowering situations, it can be difficult for the individual nurse to challenge the status quo. Eventually the individual nurse might become unable or unwilling to step outside the dominant social group and adopt whatever the dominant health care practice is within this group, which might not be health promotion (Warne and McAndrew 2004; Peel 2005). Of course, these types of findings present a bleaker picture than is often experienced – which, in the main, is not usually the case. Even where these situations present themselves in a 'mild' way, though, might be compelling enough to hold individual nurses back.

Historically, nurses have worked to improve the quality of their practice environment through research, education and political activity (Warne and McAndrew 2004).

Many hospitals and community based services have adopted more collaborative working arrangements, where nurses have greater autonomy and leadership in the provision of patient care (DoH 1999). Globally, such developments have manifested in various guises. These include Nursing Development Units in the UK (Wright 2000), whereas, in New Zealand and Australia, services have been predicated on notions of 'shared governance' (Bamford and Porter-O'Grady 2000) and, in the USA, the introduction of 'magnet hospitals' (Gifford et al. 2002). All of these examples adopt whole organizational approaches to quality improvement, humanistic approaches to caring and competence based approaches to performance management. These concepts align themselves well for promoting and supporting health promotion practice – particularly for nurses.

Nurses working in positive health care environments experience higher levels of workplace health – illustrated by gains in levels of teamwork and job satisfaction, and decreases in rates of illness, absenteeism, turnover and patient mortality (O'Brien-Pallas and Baumann 2000; Wright 2000; Whitehead 2006). These working environments can be described as health-promoting because not only do such organizations have a more informed idea of the community they serve, but they also ensure that, in meeting these needs, their employees are seen as being part of the overall community (Johnson and Baum 2001).

The WHO (1984) previously envisaged the concept of health-promoting hospitals. Such hospitals are characterized by the adoption of an emphasis on health rather than illness, in respect of both patient care and the work environment (McBride 1994; Johnson and Baum 2001; Whitehead 2005). For further details of health promoting hospitals, please refer to Chapter 5. However, such hospitals remain few and far between. Perhaps, as more nurses begin to realize a wider organizational health promotion role, this situation will change quite markedly in the future. Many hospitals continue to operate within a medical model that is focused on health problems rather than health potential. The broadening shift of nursing away from such models of care will assist greatly. In the meantime, though, often it is the organizational environment that results in social and physical barriers to nurses developing health-promoting practice (Casey 2007). These current barriers for many include:

- Lack of time due to heavy workloads
- Inadequate resources
- Disease/task orientation to care
- Lack of authority in decision-making
- Poor interpersonal relationships
- Communication difficulties
- Professional tribalism

Unfortunately, these are longstanding and consistent problems that will require some considerable effort to overcome. Thomson and Kohli (1997) reported that time and managerial support and financial assistance for courses were obstacles to health promotion practice for many nurses. This is a finding reinforced by Warne et al. (2006), who found similar concerns with nurses trying to devise integrated approaches to developing health-promoting primary care services.

Health promotion in action

Some organizational concerns have their origins in the sociological processes of becoming a nurse and, in particular, the beliefs that nurses hold as to what constitutes health and the maintenance of health. In a study carried out by Chambers and Narayanasamy (2007), several conflicting beliefs and values were revealed in the way that nurses demonstrated their understanding of health-promoting practices. For example, while some nurses revealed their awareness of the connection between a lack of money and poor diet, they also felt that, if the individual really cared about their health and well-being, they would make different choices about what they spent their money on. The same applied to smoking, exercise and so on, where often the prevailing beliefs and values were similarly contradictory.

Tutorial brief 3.2

Think about three important aspects of health promotion. On a scale of 0–10 (0 representing no confidence, 10 being fully confident), score where your confidence would be with regard to carrying out such actions. For the aspect in which you are least confident, devise a plan of action for how you might elicit support so that you can gain greater confidence.

Many nurses have seen a lack of effective education and training in health promotion as being one of the biggest barriers to developing health-promoting practice (Plews et al. 2000; Holt and Warne 2007; Piper 2008). However, and somewhat paradoxically, Macleod-Clarke and Maben (1998) explored the health promotion practices of nurses to assess their knowledge and skill following the inclusion of broader health promotion concepts in pre-registration nurse education and training (Casey 2007). Both investigations showed that, while most nurses recognized health education as 'narrower' and health promotion as 'broader', both terms still tended 'to be regarded as lifestyle related and concerned with behaviour change' (Macleod-Clarke and Maben 1998: 188). More importantly, they believed that these activities were something directed mainly at individual patients. This observation is perhaps indicative of the dissonance often seen between rhetorical role modelling and the reality of health-promoting practice (Johnson and Baum 2001).

Summary point

While the expectation of contemporary health care practice is for the nurse to engage with patients in health promotion-related activities, there remains a lack of positive mirroring within pre-registration educational programmes.

As a consequence, when taking up posts in clinical practice, often little attention is given to health promotion as an important nursing activity. Reform of health promotion content in nursing education is needed first before we will witness the beneficial knock-on effects of changing clinical practices (Whitehead 2007).

Health promotion: the nurse as a role model

There have been a number of studies that have explored the possible reasons for nurses' personal health related behaviours (Callaghan 1999; Haddad et al. 2004, Chambers and Narayanasamy 2007). Often these studies have adopted very traditional interpretations of health promotion, commonly characterized by notions of compliance with lifestyle activities – such as diet, exercise, stress management, smoking and alcohol consumption. What is evident in these studies – and often unstated – is that, as nurses, what we share with our patients is our humanity (Warne and McAndrew 2007, 2008). While our experiences might differ from others, our needs as human beings are often very similar. For example, we all desire a sense of belonging; have a need to satisfy our hunger and the need to protect ourselves against threat, whether that is emotional or physical threat. Learning to better understand and see the world from another person's perspective by engaging with that person's experiential frame of reference is crucial to effective caring. Arguably, as individuals, we are no different from the many other individuals we engage with in our everyday practice (Freshwater 2003). However, in terms of health-promoting practice, often such existential attitudes do not extend beyond notions of personal agency. This chapter, though, argues that nurses can address this by increasing their level of awareness of who they are, and how this sense of *self* is linked to patient progress and the promotion of well-being. Such an approach better enables the nurse to recognize how their own issues might impact on their perception and understanding of what the patient brings to each encounter and interaction (Barker et al. 1999; Allen 2000).

In attempting to increase self-awareness, nurses need to best understand how they have become who they are and how their own history, and that of their patients, is likely to impact unconsciously on how the nurse–patient encounter is experienced by both the patient and nurse. Values and attitudes are powerful predispositions to what behaviours are employed, in what situation, and for what effect. For the nurse, simply knowing about the need to become health-promoting will not be enough to result in this knowledge being translated into purposeful action. It is effective education and knowledge development that provides the opportunity to ensure that what is known and said is transposed into action that others will perceive as being authentic. This is particularly true for student nurses – who will also require access to experiential, interactive and inter-subjective learning opportunities for self-discovery, and an increased understanding of personal meaning. Asking students to situate themselves in relation to their practice experiences provides an opportunity for students to deconstruct their experiences safely in terms of conceptual and experiential ways of knowing (Warne and McAndrew 2008). It is through such learning activities that the opportunity to capture the emotionality of practice is created, thus enabling students to reach new understandings in terms of self and of their practice.

Engaging in self-awareness and awareness-raising activities helps, over time, to ensure that the negative aspects of professional socialization are challenged. They help ensure greater congruence between the private and public selves, and help reduce the tensions that often result from perceptions on the part of the patient of *espoused theory* versus *theory in action* on the part of the nurse. This is the difference between merely 'giving' health education advice to clients and actually offering 'empowering choice' in a more health-promoting context. Similarly, the nurse–patient relationship has the potential to provide a context in which the nurse is able to connect with the world as an individual and acknowledge all patient experience as being meaningful. At an individual level, not valuing patient experience will have implications for how effectively the nurse can or will deliver health promotion. Attending to the subjective world of another is not an easy task; for those nurses who thrive in a personal and professional paradigm characterized by feelings of competence and being in control, the long and often arduous process of promoting change in another human being can sometimes feel overwhelming. The more nurses are faced with overwhelming change, the higher the level of anxiety and the increasing use of defence mechanisms – where, for example, denial, projection and reaction formation are used instead to maintain their sense of self. For instance, the nurse who enjoys a drink of alcohol is more likely to deny a relationship between the low cost of alcohol and excessive drinking, and less inclined to engage in socio-political action aimed at policy change relating to the pricing of alcohol.

Similarly, just as patients might be reticent to make life changes in order to improve their health, nurses might also engage in defensive behaviour within their professional practice (Casey 2007). If the nurse feels insecure in addressing health promotion issues, they will try to assert competence and control through the use of their own defence mechanisms. Professional detachment, denial of personal feelings, the use of rhetoric and the pathologizing of what we do not understand are all defence mechanisms commonly adopted by health professionals (Gallop and O'Brien 2003). Indeed, defensiveness on the part of the nurse often manifests whereby illness, medical diagnosis and prescription become the critical indicators of a safe environment, thus minimizing the moral dilemma of attending to the 'notions of promoting and maintaining health' that threaten and challenge their everyday more familiar practice (Beattie 2002). The more radical notions of empowerment, community participation and socio-political action might be the threatening practices that nurses chose to avoid.

It is important that nurses gain insight and a better understanding of their own unconscious defences if they are to avoid the generation and perpetuation of negative feelings toward their role in health education and health promotion. Those actively involved in this process attend to rather than steer away from their beliefs and presuppositions, explore the world from new perspectives, develop new ways of making sense of experience and changed interpersonal attributes, and question the restraints imposed by beliefs that have been taken for granted as being true (Crowe and Luty 2005). For example, the nurse who is overweight might unconsciously deny the connection between health problems and obesity. Once they are aware of such denial, they will be better placed to explore the health-promoting activities with the patient that experiences weight related health problems. This is a crucial approach, if the objectives of health-promoting policy are to be achieved. It is through the nurse being able to recognize and explore the current context of the individual's (patient's) experience of their health status, against the socio-cultural world within which they live, that nurses have the opportunity to participate in meaning-making. This involves the nurse working with the patient to explore the patient's felt experience and the perspective this gives rise to, as well as promoting the emergence of alternative constructions. This is an approach that requires nurses to think about nursing as being not so much about caring 'for' patients as caring 'about' them, bringing an awareness of the wider determinants of health (discussed in Chapter 1) that contribute to, in this case, say, obesity.

Summary point

Nursing is an inter-subjective activity, in that it involves the coming together of two or more people who are shaped by their own history, culture, beliefs and values – some of which is unconscious. If health promotion is to be successful, it requires the nurse to bring to consciousness these aspects of self and the way in which they influence and impact on interpersonal relationships with patients. In reconceptualizing self, and self in relation to others, the nurse will be able to form new and more meaningful perspectives.

 ### Tutorial brief 3.3

Think about two aspects of your own health and well-being that could be improved through using health promotion strategies. Reflect on what factors might have prevented you addressing these aspects in your own life. Consider how the same or similar factors might have been applicable to patients you have engaged with in health promotion activities. If you were to address these for yourself, identify the sources of evidence that would be effective in helping achieve this goal. Having considered the lifestyle choices you have made in terms of the impact upon your health and well-being, reflect on the extent of any moral imperative to ask others to 'do as I say and not as I do'.

Health promotion: some practical steps

This chapter argues that if nurses are going to be able to turn a healthy rhetoric into a healthy reality, health-promoting ways of *being* and *doing* must be actualized, perhaps in this context through some form of *action learning*. Typically, action learning involves a group of people finding ways to test and evaluate theory in a real-life context, using a cycle of action and reflection to produce self-determined change (Clark 2000). This is an approach that reflects the fundamental principles of developing health-promoting practice; that is, adopting an approach that is predicated on doing '*with*' rather than '*for*' people for whom any change is intended, (Clark 2000). In other words, it requires acknowledgement of self-empowerment, community empowerment and socio-political action. If, as a nurse, you are currently involved in activities that allows for a better understanding of the barriers to health promotion practice, you will be in a better position to deal with these barriers. If you then do this within a group, the creativity and problem-solving opportunities will be increased. This is an approach that helps to ensure a shared commitment to becoming health-promoting practitioners through achieving ownership of the problems and solutions. Many of the organizational barriers already noted can be tackled by the action learning group of nurses in a way that reflects their particular organizational circumstances, thus making outcomes easier to implement (Clark 2000). Action learning approaches can start to facilitate a shared approach to the development of health-promoting practice at an organizational level – but it is also an effective way for providing a safe learning opportunity for you as an individual to become more aware of who you are, your beliefs, attitudes and values, and how these are used in relationships with others. Perhaps the following exercise might elaborate on this:

 Tutorial brief 3.4

Think about three patients you have worked with in your clinical practice and identify what the presenting health needs were. Now, consider each of those people with regard to their socio-economic and cultural contexts, and how these might have impacted on their health problem. Taking all these factors into account, develop a *health promotion strategy* for each of these people. In developing your strategies, consideration needs to be given to: the additional knowledge you might need to undertake this task, skills you need to develop in order to be competent in promoting health, opportunities for maximizing health promotion for each person, information that you would share with each person, and identification of what could be done at a macro (organizational) level to improve each of these particular health problems.

Once you have worked through the above exercise for yourself, you could present your thinking and outcomes to other colleagues. This point in the action learning process is always the most difficult. Try to approach it with an open mind and an awareness that your unconscious self will already be preparing to use a defence mechanism against whatever it is your colleagues might have to say about your thinking. Learning, and the subsequent development of a more health-promoting form of practice, will be best achieved in acknowledging these defence processes and enlisting the help of your colleagues in better understanding why you might be employing them in relation to what you are presenting.

Conclusion

This chapter has explored the relationship between the individual (the nurse), the profession, (nursing) and the context within which nursing occurs (the organization). A number of personal, professional and organizational factors were identified that either enhance or inhibit the provision of health-promoting activities. These included the pervasive and potent forces of socialization into a profession where, largely, the preparation for practice is predicated on illness models; organizational imperatives and how these are experienced as the busyness of every day practice; and perceived lack of education on promoting evidence based approaches to achieving well-being. It was noted that, in the same way that many individuals will resist health educational messages, nurses will – either by omission or decision – not engage in health promoting activities that might stand as role models or educational examples of good practice. The reason for this is often complex and might not even be a response of which the individual is aware. While many nurses generally believe that health promotion is an important part of their work, this belief often only exists at a rhetorical level. The reality can be different. There is a need for nurse educators to work more closely in ensuring greater congruence between espoused theory and theory in use. Such closer working needs to be underpinned by a lifelong curriculum capable of facilitating inter-professional learning to enable nursing staff to acquire the knowledge and skills for health promotion practice. Nurses are potential catalysts for change in current health promotion practice. To fulfil this potential, continued dialogue between those that commission practice and educational provision needs to be focused on the preparation of future nurses, so they are able to work confidently with 'up-stream' health-promoting initiatives, rather than continuing only to engage in effectively meeting illness driven demands for health care services.

Summary point

In keeping with contemporary policy, nurses need to give careful consideration to how they are able to integrate health-promoting activities into their everyday practice, and what organizational, professional and personal factors might hinder this process.

Additional resources

Bradford M. and Whinn S. (1997) 'Practice Nursing and Health Promotion: A Case Study', in Sidell, M., Jones, L., Katz, J. and Peberdy, A. (eds), *Debates and Dilemmas in Promoting Health: A Reader* (Oxford: Open University/Macmillan Press).

Piper S. (2008) 'A Qualitative Study Exploring the Relationship between Nursing and Health Promotion Language, Theory and Practice', *Nurse Education Today*, 28: 186–93.

Whitehead D. (2005) 'The Culture, Context and Progress of Health Promotion in Nursing', in Scriven A. (ed.), *Health Promoting Practice: The Contribution of Nurses and Allied Health Professionals* (London: Palgrave Macmillan).

References

Allen, D. (2000) '"I'll tell you what suits me best if you don't mind me saying": Lay Participation in Health Care', *Nursing Inquiry*, 7: 182–90.

Bamford, A. and Porter-O'Grady, T. (2000) 'Shared Governance within the Market-oriented System of New Zealand', *International Nursing Review*, 47: 83–8.

Barker, P., Jackson, S. and Stevenson, C. (1999) 'What are Psychiatric Nurses Needed For? Developing a Theory of Essential Nursing Practice', *Journal of Psychiatric and Mental Health Nursing*, 6: 273–82.

Baumann, A., O'Brien-Pallas, L. and Armstrong-Stassen, M. (2001) *Commitment and Care: The Benefits of a Healthy Workplace for Nurses, Their Patients and the System (A Policy Synthesis)* (Ottowa: Canadian Health Services Research Foundation/Change Foundation).

Beattie, A. (2002) 'Education for Systems Change: A Key Resource for Radical Action on Health', in Adams, L., Amos, M. and Munro, J. (eds), *Promoting Health: Politics and Practice* (London: Sage).

Borchardt, G. (2000) 'Role Models for Health Promotion: The Challenge for Nurses', *Nursing Forum*, 35: 29–32.

Buresh, B. and Gordon, S. (2000) *From Silence to Voice: What Nurses Know and Must Communicate to the Public* (Ottowa: Canadian Nurses Association).

Callaghan, P. (1999) 'Health Beliefs and their Influence on United Kingdom Nurses' Health-related Behaviours', *Journal of Advanced Nursing*, 29: 28–35.

Carlson, G. and Warne, T. (2007) 'Do Healthier Nurses make Better Health Promoters? A Review of the Literature', *Nurse Education Today*, 27: 506–13.

Carr, G. (2008) 'Changes in Nurse Education: Delivering the Curriculum', *Nurse Education Today*, 28(1), January: 120–7.

Casey, D. (2007) 'Nurses' Perceptions, Understanding and Experiences of Health Promotion', *Journal of Clinical Nursing*, 16: 1039–49.

Chambers, D. and Narayanasamy, A. (2007) 'A Discourse and Foucauldian Analysis of Nurses' Health Beliefs: Implications for Nurse Education', *Nurse Education Today*, 28: 155–62.

Clark, J.E. (2000) 'Action Research', in Cormack, D. (ed.), *The Research Process in Nursing*, 4th edn (Oxford: Blackwell Science).

Clark, E., McCann, T., Rowe, K. and Lazenbatt, A. (2003) 'Cognitive Dissonance and Undergraduate Nursing Students' Knowledge of, and Attitudes about, Smoking', *Journal of Advanced Nursing*, 46(6): 586–94.

Crowe, M. and Luty, S. (2005) 'Interpersonal Psychotherapy: An Effective Psychotherapeutic Intervention for Mental Health Nursing Practice', *International Journal of Mental Health Nursing*, 14: 24–31.

DoH (1999) *Making a Difference: Strengthening the Nursing, Midwifery and Health Visiting Contribution to Health and Health Care* (London: HMSO, Department of Health).

DoH (2004) *Choosing Health: Partial Public Sector Impact Assessment. Supporting NHS Front Line Staff in Health Improvement*, Annex 5 (London: HMSO, Department of Health).

DoH (2006) *Our Health, Our Care, Our Say* (London: HMSO, Department of Health).

Freshwater, D. (2003) *Therapeutic Nursing: Improving Patient Care through Self Awareness and Reflection* (London: Sage).

Gallop, R. and O'Brien, L. (2003) 'Re-Establishing Psychodynamic Theory as Foundational Knowledge for Psychiatric/Mental Health Nursing', *Issues in Mental Health Nursing*, 24: 213–27.

Gifford, B., Zammuto, R., Goodman, E. and Hill, K. (2002) 'The Relationship between Hospital Unit Culture and Nurses' Quality of Work Life: Practitioner Application', *Journal of Healthcare Management*, 47(1): 13–26.

Haddad, L., Kane, D., Rajacich, D., Cameron, S. and Al-Ma'aitah, R. (2004) 'A Comparison of Health Practices of Canadian and Jordanian Nursing Students', *Public Health Nursing*, 21: 85–90.

Holt, M. and Warne, T. (2007) 'Pushing at an Open or Closed Door: Training Pre-Registration Student Nurses as Future Health Promoters', *Nurse Education in Practice*, 7: 373–80.

ICN (2000) *Nursing Matters: ICN on Mobilising Nurses for Health Promotion* (Geneva: ICN).

Johnson, A. and Baum, F. (2001) 'Health Promotion Hospitals: A Typology of Different Organisational Approaches to Health Promotion', *Health Promotion International*, 16: 281–7.

Jordan, S. (2000) 'Educational Input and Patient Outcomes: Exploring the Gap', *Journal of Advanced Nursing*, 31: 461–71.

Latter, S. and Westwood, G. (2001) *Public Health Capacity in the Nursing Workforce. Phase 1: A Pilot Project to Identify Current Practice in Educational Preparation* (Southampton: University of Southampton, School of Nursing and Midwifery).

Macleod-Clarke, J. and Maben, J. (1998) 'Health Promotion: Perceptions of Project 2000 Educated Nurses', *Health Education Research*, 13: 185–96.

McBride, A. (1994) 'Health Promotion in Hospitals: The Attitudes, Beliefs and Practices of Hospital Nurses', *Journal of Advanced Nursing*, 20: 92–100.

McCann, T., Clark, E. and Rowe, K. (2005) 'Undergraduate Nursing Students' Attitudes towards Smoking Health Promotion', *Nursing and Health Sciences*, 7, 164–74.

Norton, L. (1998) 'Health Promotion and Health Education: What Role should the Nurse Adopt in Practice?, *Journal of Advanced Nursing*, 28: 1269–75.

O'Brien-Pallas, L. and Baumann, A. (2000) 'Toward Evidence Based Policy Decisions: A Case Study of Nursing Health Human Resources in Ontario, Canada', *Nursing Inquiry*, 7: 248–57.

Olshansky, E. (2007) 'Nurses and Health Promotion', *Journal of Professional Nursing*, 23: 1–2.

Peel, D. (2005) 'Dual Professionalism: Facing the Challenges of Continuing Professional Development in the Work Place', *Reflective Practice*, 6: 123–40.

Piper, S. (2008) 'A Qualitative Study exploring the relationship between Nursing and Health Promotion Language, Theory and Practice', *Nurse Education Today*, 28: 186–93.

Plews, C., Billingham, K. and Rowe, A. (2000) 'Public Health Nursing: Barriers and Opportunities', *Health and Social Care in the Community*, 8: 138–46.

RCN (2007) *Nurses as Partners in delivering Public Health* (London: RCN).

Rush, K. (2002) *Self as Role Model in Health Promotion: Development of an Empirical Instrument*, PhD, Georgia State University (Ann Arbor, MI: UMI).

Rutherford, J., Leigh, J., Monk, J. and Murray, C. (2005) 'Creating an Organizational Infrastructure to Develop and Support New Nursing Roles – A Framework for Debate', *Journal of Nursing Management*, 13: 97–105.

Scriven, A. and Garman, S. (eds) (2005) *Promoting Health: Global Perspectives* (Basingstoke: Palgrave Macmillan).

Shamian, J. (2005) 'Be True to Yourself and Your Values', *Canadian Journal of Nurse Leadership*, 18: 19–22.

Stokols, D., Allen, J. and Bellingham, R. (1996) 'The Social Ecology of Health Promotion: Implications for Research and Practice', *American Journal of Health Promotion*, 10: 247–51.

Thomson, P. and Kohli, H. (1997) 'Health Promotion Training Needs Analysis: An Integral Role for Clinical Nurses in Lanarkshire, Scotland', *Journal of Advanced Nursing*, 26: 507–14.

Warne, T., King, M., Street, C. and McAlonan, C. (2006) *Finding the Evidence for Education and Training to Deliver Integrated Health and Social Care: The Primary Care Workforce Perspective*, Shaping the Future for Primary Care Education and Training Project, University of Salford.

Warne, T. and McAndrew, S. (2004) Nursing, Nurse Education and Professionalisation in a Contemporary Context', in Warne, T. and McAndrew, S. (eds), *Using Patient Experience in Nurse Education* (Basingstoke: Palgrave).

Warne, T. and McAndrew, S. (2007) 'Passive Patient or Engaged Expert? Using a Ptolemaic Approach to Enhance Mental Health Nurse Education and Practice', *International Journal of Mental Health Nursing*, 16: 224–9.

Warne, T. and McAndrew, S. (2008) 'Painting the Landscape of Emotionality: Colouring in the Emotional Gaps between the Theory and Practice of Mental Health Nursing', *International Journal of Mental Health Nursing*, 17(2), April: 108–15.

Watson, J. (2006) '"Can an Ethic of Caring be maintained?", 30th anniversary invited editorial reflecting on law, Harrison, L. (1990)', *Maintaining the Ethic of Caring in Nursing*', *Journal of Advanced Nursing*, 54: 257–9.

Whitehead, D. (2005) Health Promoting Hospitals: The Role and Function of Nursing', *Journal of Clinical Nursing*, 14: 20–7.

Whitehead, D. (2006) 'Workplace Health Promotion: The Role and Responsibilities of Health Care Managers', *Journal of Nursing Management*, 14, 59–68.

Whitehead, D. (2007) 'Reviewing Health Promotion in Nursing Education', *Nurse Education Today*, 27: 225–37.

Wright, S. (2000) 'Picking Up the Pieces', *Australian Journal of Holistic Nursing*, 7: 9–12.

WHO (1984) *Health Promotion: A Discussion Document on Concepts and Principles* (Copenhagen: WHO, Regional Office for Europe).

WHO (2000) *Nurse and Midwives for Health: A WHO European Strategy for Nursing and Midwifery Education* (Copenhagen: WHO, Regional Office for Europe).

CHAPTER 4

A Systematic Approach to Health Promotion

Dean Whitehead

Objectives

By the end of this chapter you should be able to:

- Identify what constitutes a systematic approach to health promotion
- Examine what processes make up a systematic approach to health promotion – that is, assessment, planning and evaluation
- Determine popular existing frameworks for guiding health promotion practice
- Identify what constitutes a systematic approach to health education
- Acknowledge the contribution of evidence-based practice to systematic approaches

---

Key terms
- Assessing health promotion
- Evaluating health promotion
- Evidence based practice
- Health promotion process
- Planning health promotion

Introduction

Health promotion is a dynamic and often complex process that cannot be applied in a haphazard manner. It mostly fails where there is little or no attempt to incorporate well-structured and systematic process. It is well established that the more systematic and structured our health promotion activities are, the more likely that they will be both effective and efficient (Tones and Tilford 2001; Nutbeam and

Wise 2004). One of the criticisms justifiably aimed at many health professionals' health promotion practice, however, is that they often fail to incorporate such processes into their practice. Many health promotion interventions are therefore criticized for being unstructured, opportunistic, *ad hoc* and failing to comply with established systematic processes. It would appear, then, that health promotion practice might not be appropriately planned, assessed, measured or evaluated. These are essential parts of the overall process of effective health promotion practice, and nurses are becoming adept at incorporating effective and structured processes into their health promotion practice.

Adherence to the *overall* process of health promotion is vital. There are a number of examples in the nursing literature where elements of good health promotion practice are demonstrated (for example, Nuñez et al. 2003; Liu et al. 2006). However, sometimes, examples might still be criticized for only incorporating elements of the overall process instead of all of the identified components. For instance, it is well documented that, while many health promoters plan their activities well, they often fail to evaluate their interventions for outcome and effectiveness (Tones and Tilford 2001; Naidoo and Wills 2000; Wills 2007).

More than ten years ago, Thomson (1998) described the fact that many nurses were inclined to practice their health related interventions on the basis of chance, rather than on proven or planned need. These health promotion encounters subsequently did not always result in their intended outcomes, whether the outcomes were formally identified or not. Sentiments such as this helped to draw attention to the need to make health related programmes and interventions as focused and directed as possible – and this development is more notable in the nursing literature today. This chapter aims to describe and explore good practice as it applies to all of the essential health promotion elements required to demonstrate effective process. It does so by presenting these in a logical and sequential order, and offers models and frameworks for guiding this type of process. From this position, it is intended that all nurses can adopt and adapt this information as part of a positive contribution to their health promotion practice.

The 'overall' process of health promotion

Before viewing overall health promotion process, it is useful to identify some of the popular contemporary health promotion theories and models. Some are more effective or useful than others for guiding the health promotion process. For instance, several contemporary models are useful for demonstrating the nature and intention of health promotion, but they are more about highlighting what health promotion looks like and, therefore, less concerned with structured implementation. These contemporary models offer theoretical frameworks that help to facilitate an appreciation of the health promotion process but, less so, they impact less directly on clinical practice. This is true of the Triphasic Map of Health Education (French and Adams 1986), the Four Paradigms of Health Promotion (Caplan and Holland 1990), the Strategies of Health Promotion (Beattie 1991) and Tannahill's Typology of Health Promotion (Downie et al. 1996). Some authors, when describing the health promotion process, might also really be referring to socio-cognitive behavioural models – for example, Becker's (1974) Health Belief Model (incorporating Bandura's elaborations on self-efficacy), Azjen and Fishbein's (1980) Theory of Reasoned Action Model, Prochaska and DiClemente's (1984) Revolving Door Model and Tones' Health Action Model (1987) and so on. For fuller explanations of these models, see Whitehead (2001a) and Chapter 1. These socio-cognitive behavioural models are mentioned later in this chapter, too. While these models are often useful to consider as part of a health promotion programme, they are mostly centred on individualized behavioural change theories. These theories are more consistent with *health education* processes (see Chapter 1). Nurses might relate to these theories more in terms of the health information that is often offered to people during their in-patient hospital/clinic stays –either to alleviate ongoing effects of existing disease or to offset the risk of potential onset of disease. Today, health promotion frameworks and models are more appropriately considered alongside community and population health interventions. These interventions might or might not include the behavioural theories and models mentioned above.

Additional point

While community based models are the most appropriate for organizing health promotion programmes, this does not mean that they cannot be used by nurses based in acute or institutional settings. These types of establishments should be viewed as part of the community and not separate from it. Effective hospitals, clinics and so on offer 'seamless services' whereby health promotion activities occur within these settings and link, through multi-disciplinary and multi-agency referral and collaboration, beyond their walls and boundaries and into the hearts and homes of clients in their own living environments.

 ### Tutorial brief 4.1

Try to access further information about the theoretical and socio-cognitive models by making Internet searches of academic databases – for example, GoogleScholar. Can you identify the strengths and limitations of these models as examples of theoretical frameworks that could potentially influence your health promotion practice and process? For instance, under what circumstances does their behavioural focus assist nursing practice, and where might this focus limit practice?

Chapter 2 has already described the theoretical and philosophical positions that underpin the various theories and philosophies of health promotion process. According to Tones (2000: 229),

> To critically evaluate the effectiveness and efficiency of any [health promotion] programme which is theoretically and methodologically unsound is either naïve or cynical and certainly renders a major disservice to health promotion.

Research, however, shows that these positions are not always translated into practice (Wise and Signal 2000). Berentson-Shaw and Price (2007) inform us that the real challenge is to find ways for these theoretical positions to be fully integrated into health promotion practice, so that their activities contribute effectively to population health gain. The most useful way to ensure that this happens is by critically reviewing and breaking down the processes of health promotion into its constituent parts. Before this chapter addresses this and explores each process in turn, it is necessary to view the process as a whole by exploring a few of the most widely used contemporary health promotion process models.

Flowchart for Planning and Evaluating Health Promotion Model

One of the more popular contemporary planning models is Ewles and Simnett's (2003) Flowchart for Planning and Evaluating Health Promotion Model. It is a generalized model that is popular for its ease of use. The flowchart breaks down the overall health promotion process into a series of linear stepped stages that are closely related to each other and cyclical in nature. The self-explanatory stages begin with identifying needs and priorities, setting aims and objectives, best aims, identifying resources, planning evaluation methods and setting action plans – all leading to the final ACTION stage (which includes implementation of plan and evaluation). The content of this chapter follows a similar order, as this type of sequential process is the 'natural order' of any well thought through health promotion programme. For this reason, the Ewles and Simnett (2003) model is not fully detailed here, as its stages are elaborated on further in the following sections of this chapter.

One of the criticisms of the Ewles and Simnett model is that, while easier for those in the early stages of health promotion to incorporate into their nursing practice, it might not adequately serve the needs of more complex health promotion programmes. From this point of view, one of the most popular wider-reaching contemporary health promotion models is the Precede-Proceed model.

The Precede-Proceed model

The Precede-Proceed model of health programme planning and evaluation builds on more than forty years' work by Lawrence W. Green and colleagues, and was first published in 1980. The model was adapted and built upon each time a new edition of *Health Promotion Planning* was published, and is now in its fourth edition (2005). The original Precede model was a rather crude four-phase model that drew from the fields of epidemiology, social-cognitive psychology (behavioural diagnosis), education, and management (administrative diagnosis). Its main limitation was that it was a linear, causal-chain planning model that focused on behavioural aspects of health, rather than the wider health promotion strategies that are more common today. The Precede model, where it is used on its own, is more likely to be adopted for *health education* programmes than wider-reaching health promotion activities. It is worth noting that, despite its complexity, the popularity of the Precede model meant that it has been revised by others, such as Bonaguro and Miaoulis, who have adapted it to incorporate a broader 'social marketing' approach to their health strategies (Whitehead 2000).

In collaboration with Marshall Kreuter, the second edition of *Health Promotion Planning* extended the Precede model to incorporate wider ecological, environmental, policy, organizational and social determinants of health. These were factors that Green and Kreuter had subsequently found important while they were engaged in national community health promotion programmes (Green and Kreuter 1991, 1992). This introduced the Proceed phase of the revised original Precede model.

In their third edition, Green and Kreuter added further dimensions of health programming (Green and Kreuter 1999). Figure 4.1 shows the third edition of the

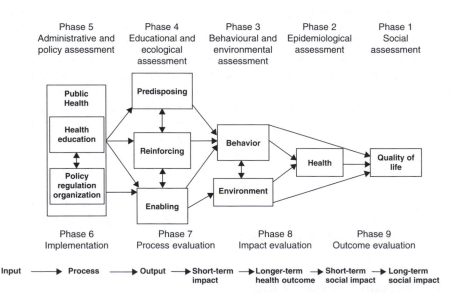

Figure 4.1 Surveillance, planning and evaluation for policy and action: precede–proceed model
Source: Green and Kreuter (1999) reproduced with the permission of The McGraw-Hill Companies.

Precede-Proceed model. This adaptation made the model even more health promoting in its scope, yet also had the effect of making it more complex to use. The original authors have acknowledged this, and so the fourth edition has attempted to simplify the process (Green and Kreuter 2005). Green and Kreuter's (2005) current thinking on health promotion planning advocates a socio-ecological process with an emphasis on community partnership, and a converging systematic, integrative framework for practice (Kreuter et al. 2004; Green and Kreuter 2005).

The popularity and use of the Precede-Proceed model has never been in question. The third edition of the model alone has been applied, tested, adapted and verified in over 960 published studies over the last decade or more. Some useful examples of its process are highlighted in studies by the likes of McGhan et al. (2002) and Chiang (2003). Following the third edition, a survey of 253 universities offering graduate or undergraduate degree specialization in health promotion reported that the Precede-Proceed model was taught by 88 per cent of respondents, used by 85.7 per cent in teaching, and used by 74.6 per cent in practice – the most among the top 10 health promotion planning models listed (Linnan et al. 2005). The respondents also ranked Precede-Proceed highest among the 10 planning models on usefulness for research (86 per cent) and usefulness for practice (90.8 per cent). These figures suggest that nurses would be well advised at least to consider such a model before framing their health promotion strategies. A website exists devoted to the Precede-Proceed model (http://www.lgreen.net). It is on this website that the modified and simplified fourth edition revision of the Precede-Proceed model can be viewed (http://www.lgreen.net/precede.htm).

Health promotion in action

Savelson et al. (2005) report on how an adapted form of the Precede-Proceed model emerged from their community based sustainability planning project. This was a five-year project designed to investigate how citizens of the Georgia Basin region of British Columbia could learn, over the next forty years, to live within the limits of natural ecosystems while improving overall well-being. This was identified as a means of achieving a sustainable health related future for the region. By guiding the researchers and citizens through a process of prioritization, the Precede-Proceed model assisted in identifying the measures needed to best address raised concerns and issues. As a result of this process, priorities such as an affordable housing strategy were implemented.

Summary point

There are many frameworks and models that can be adopted with health promotion interventions. Many, however, are adaptations of several contemporary models – with perhaps the most recognized being the Precede-Proceed model.

Tutorial brief 4.2

Imagine that you wanted to consider the 'whole' process of a health promotion intervention, prior to commencing the process in your nursing practice. Before reading on, what factors do you think would need to be in place? Make a list of them.

Assessing health promotion

A lack of structured assessment and planning will invariably result in ineffective health promotion interventions, since they are initial and vital parts of the whole process of health promotion and community development. Pender et al. (2006) confirm that community assessment is performed as a primary building block for the planning, implementation and evaluation of health promotion programmes. While this chapter separates the two processes of assessment and planning they are, in reality, very closely inter-related. For some, it can be difficult to determine where the assessment stage ends and the planning phase begins. With some programmes the activities will occur at the same time. Poor attention to either of the processes, though, will inevitably lead to poor implementation in practice. It is essential, therefore, that the nurse pays particular attention to how they go about their health promotion activities; namely, through the initial processes of assessment and planning. The planning process is explored later in this chapter.

Additional point

For some, the term 'assessment' is similar to 'evaluation' – that is, to assess something is to identify if it works or not. In this case though, assessment is the initial process whereby a nurse would be looking at the viability of conducting health promotion prior to implementation.

The first stage of conducting a health promotion intervention lies with the assessment phase. This represents the preliminary investigation into the feasibility, efficacy and acceptability of any intervention involving clients in their health settings. Nurses need to know who to target, how accessible these groups and individuals are to them, the overall health priorities of the community, and the resources (both human and structural) that are available and can be readily mobilized. An initial assessment of community willingness, cooperation and opportunity (both of the community members and of the nurses and other health professionals involved) is required in order to assess community capacity for health promotion action and change. Nurses, as well as focusing on the capability of the immediate community being assessed, will also have to assess their own capacity and ability to act and perform in a variety of settings (Gandelman et al. 2006). Community members will be more confident in the abilities of nurses who they deem are capable, well prepared and who offer appropriately constructed interventions.

For an effective health promotion assessment to be completed, a *community assessment* is required, accompanied by *needs assessment* process. A community assessment is a comprehensive description of the overall health needs of a population (community) and the already existing resources to facilitate this need. Nurses wishing to know what currently helps or hinders a whole community to influence its overall health needs would find this information useful. Needs assessment traditionally identifies the health needs of specific groups within a targeted population. It assesses what is currently being done to meet those needs, and what programmes and services (existing and needed) should be prioritized (Peterson and Alexander 2001). Nurses would conduct this type of assessment where they wanted to explore the potential feasibility of setting up specific health services – for example, diabetes clinics in a high-risk population area. Both of the described assessment processes require the active participation and voice of the targeted population in identifying their health priorities and as a means of developing a realistic plan of future action. As McMurray (2007: 76) states:

> Communities are inherently social organizations and community residents are instrumental in shaping community dynamics and cohesion – both vital for engaging communities in health promotion.

Seeking individual and overall community opinion is therefore needed for a successful outcome.

Health promotion in action

Aponte and Nickitas (2007) describe their collaborative nurse led health promotion programme to address health disparities in an urban underserved community. Part of their assessment strategy involved a needs assessment of the local population that resulted in a health fair being organized as a vehicle to meet and inform local residents on currently available health care systems and resources that they could access.

Many targeted communities will often present with a higher degree of disadvantage compared with nearby or surrounding communities. Health priorities will often centre on the structural issues that act as barriers to good health – for example, crime, pollution, lack of health facilities, poor education, poor standards of housing and so on. Health priorities might centre on specific diseases, and especially those that are directly linked to environmental issues. For example, this could be where asthma is associated with poor air quality and housing problems. However, traditional health related programmes that target the consequences and management of disease related states alone are known to be ineffective in many cases. Where they are useful is when they are used alongside health promotion activities that also act on and alter the wider structural determinants of disease-causing states. For instance, nurses working with asthma clients also assess for the most likely environmental trigger factors and then seek to educate on how they can be avoided, and what policies and resources are in place to support this. As Gomm et al. (2006: 284) state:

> Hence, contemporary public health practice [health promotion] involves not only attempting to change individual behaviour but also influencing the policies and practices that create the conditions for change.

In other words this is a preventative approach to health related practice.

Health promotion in action

Gandelman et al. (2006) describe how assessment activities assist with community intervention HIV prevention, and how they have particularly helped health promotion programmes in California and Denver, USA. Although the focus is on a disease specific state, the intention was to explore how highly structured assessment processes assist with whole community capacity in dealing with the issues raised by and affecting entire populations.

Additional point

Community needs assessment is a very broad process that will also be accompanied by *group needs assessment* and *individual needs assessment*. What is known, though, is that the more individualized the assessment becomes, the greater the likelihood of it adopting more personalized behavioural-change forms of health education management.

Tutorial brief 4.3

When performing needs assessments, we should be aware that there are several different forms of need, all of which require assessment. They are 'felt need', 'expressed need', 'normative need' and 'comparative need'. Define each type of need and identify how nurses might assess that form of need, and for what reasons.

Why do we need to assess health promotion?

According to MacDonald (1998: 188):

> Any health promotion initiative, be it for an individual or for an entire community, has a specific and definable aim. It is itself made up of a series of assessable components [that ensures that] ... the target problem is being addressed.

Where nurses seek the effective assessment of the appropriateness of a community based health promotion intervention, they are advised not to 'go in blind'. Instead, through assessment, they are able to separate problems from solutions and are better able to set priorities for action. This separation ensures that activities have been well thought through – which pays dividends, especially when difficulties crop up that had not previously been considered or encountered. This is not just relevant to community based interventions; careful assessment is equally important for acute based interventions. A further consideration is that, where nurses are working in disadvantaged communities, they are unlikely to be part of that community – except by professional association. That is not always the case, though. For instance, there are examples in New Zealand of Maori nurse practitioners (with prescribing rights) who are specifically supported to work as the lead health promotion professional in the heart of the high health need Maori dominated communities. Arrangements that enable nurses to assess situations alongside integral members of that community will help to facilitate sympathetic, culturally grounded and well-informed endeavours. Where nurses might belong to a different cultural group than the community in which they seek to work, it is still vital to ensure 'culturally competent and safe' practices. In this case, nurses would ideally have some identifiable link or association with that community or, alternatively, be well versed in its underpinning cultural values and practices.

Summary point

Cultural considerations are an important aspect of health promotion nursing assessment. How would you, as a nurse, orientate yourself to a cultural population that was different to yours?

Community needs assessment is not just involved with a local needs assessment process but also includes *asset based assessment* (Gandelman et al. 2006). This type of assessment allows nurses insight into what immediate resources are available to aid population health and, at the same time, allows for mapping of what is *not* in place. Another important consideration is that assessment activities benefit the health promotion process in the beginning stages, and also help to inform the selection and adaptation of a health promotion programme over time.

Health promotion in action

Nuñez et al. (2003) report on the successful nurse managed Escalante Health Partnership health promotion programme – providing wellness services for a suburban, multi-generational, multi-ethnic, lower socio-economic status community in Arizona, USA. They report that this partnership has developed into a dynamic university–community partnership practice model that involves all local community organizations in programme assessment and planning. This offers high quality health promotion through the strength and commitment of collaborating partners and active negotiation of the affected community members.

 Tutorial brief 4.4

You want to assess your local community at large to investigate its overall health status. List what factors you might want to assess to get a clear overall picture of that community.

How do we assess health promotion?

There is a great deal of literature that contests the nature and definition of 'community' as a term in itself (see Jackson 2007). The readers of this chapter will probably already have a clear concept of what community means to them, both at a social and professional level. What a community is, and is not, does not need to be discussed here. However, the notion of *community profile* does. Without a clear and comprehensive profiling, community assessment is incomplete and it is difficult to get to the heart of health related issues or know where to begin in terms of approaching issues, resources or people. A community profile should ideally be the first stage of a community assessment. It is the initial stage that assists in presenting the 'overall picture' of a specific community. In essence, nurses require at least a 'snapshot' of whatever health situation or community it is in which they are interested. Pender et al. (2006) suggest that this process is better viewed as a 'familiarization' assessment – providing a broad, rather than in-depth, view of the community at large. They stress that in-depth assessment, including primary and data documentation collection and analysis (epidemiological (health status) data), is best reserved for situations where it is absolutely essential compared with high priority programme goals. Jackson (2007) identifies that there are three broad approaches to assessing community need:

- *Epidemiological approach*, which uses factual data on health and illness trends in a community. When nurses access health statistics and details of health trends, especially in relation to mortality and morbidity rates, these data are likely to be epidemiological in nature.

- *Corporate or stakeholder approach*, in which key agencies, service providers and health professionals are asked about population based health issues. For this part of community need, nurses will liaise with a wide range of health agencies.
- *Individual approach*, which is used as the process of determining both the community's and individual community members' feelings about the most pressing needs, and how to address them. This requires nurses to participate in active face-to-face contact with those most in need of health services provision.

The first two positions tend to be 'expert led' and are directed by health professionals – such as nurses, themselves. The third, community-driven approach is one that Jackson (2007) believes to be the most neglected of the three approaches, and yet it is the most appropriate approach for community development programmes because it directly engages the community according to their own priorities.

A community profile would primarily be nurse driven, but it is always advisable to seek the information from community members themselves. There is some blurring between the similar processes of a community profile compared with a *community survey*. A community survey actually compels both parties to work together. Wass (2000) lists what topics should be observed and measured in a community profile. They are:

- History of the community – both past and recent
- General environment
- Nature of residents
- Types of organizations
- Communication methods and structures
- Where the seats of power and leadership lie

There is a range of processes, both simple and complex, for assessing community needs. At the simplest level, Wass (2000) helpfully breaks down the types of activities that assist in promoting a broad, yet comprehensive and insightful assessment of community. They are:

- Listening to and taking notice of the community
- Assessing local social and economic indicators
- Drawing upon epidemiological data – but also realizing its limitations and so striving for broader approaches to health assessment
- Seeking the views of health professionals and other professionals who work within the assessed community
- Reviewing state, regional or national policies – especially those emerging from community consultation

Similarly, McMurray (2007) identifies a useful initial framework for assessing health promotion interventions. She advocates a five-step plan that involves:

- Generally observing and measuring 'the lay of the land'
- Mapping resources
- Identifying players who could/would help and assist

- Identifying structural factors already in place – that is, human resources, health systems, gatekeepers, locations and so on
- Performing a current strengths, weaknesses, opportunities and threats (SWOT) analysis of the community and its people

Pender et al. (2006) further elaborate on different sub-sets of health promotion assessment process. They detail these as:

- *Problem-orientated assessment*, where the process begins with a single problem, such as neighbourhood crime, and identifies the types of factors and resources that either assist or impede current situations
- *Sub-system assessment*, in which an in-depth assessment of a particular sector of the community of interest is undertaken

There are also many different ways of capturing assessment data including interviews, survey questionnaires, focus groups, storytelling and screening (Jackson 2007). Nurses are necessarily required to be conversant with a range of health assessment techniques, but this does not have to be too complex. Being familiar with a small range of appropriate techniques – but techniques that are well understood by the nurse or other colleagues with whom they are working – will suffice.

With health promotion assessment, it is the initial exploration of place, structures and resources that should produce a general picture of the types of health promotion interventions that are potentially possible, desirable and measurable. This is all conducted before leading onto the next stage of the process – that of planning. An assessment of a client or community does not merely represent the means to determine a health status position; it is also the beginning of the planning process that needs to be applied to any health intervention for it to be effective.

Additional point

With health promotion assessment it is actually best to start with a 'blank sheet' perspective. Until nurses have conducted the preliminary assessment of the targeted population and discussed health issues, needs and priorities with members of this community, the course of action required should be regarded as unknown. To act in any other way runs the risk of subjective and assumptive assessment.

Summary point

Assessment is a vital first stage component of the health promotion process. Community and needs based assessment must actively involve all key stakeholders for that targeted community, especially key members of that community.

Planning health promotion

The next step on from assessment is the planning phase, which entails working out how the assessment findings can be put into place where appropriate. Once the viability of a health promotion programme is established following on from effective assessment, the planning of the frameworks, structures and resources that need to be in place is the next important part of the overall process.

Health promotion planning models are specifically designed to identify and signpost the necessary step-by-step sequential stages and phases within a health promotion/health education programme. This ensures that the nurse is provided with an overview of the main issues that require attention. It also ensures that these issues are dealt with on a systematic basis and that a checklist is available during the planning process. In essence, planning models assist with the development of effective health promotion programmes and appropriate use of resources by regularly monitoring progress throughout. This benefits nursing practice because regular scrutiny allows mistakes to be noted and acted on, and successes to be built on. Planning models are particularly useful because they also 'force' nurses to address the realities and logistics of conducting health programmes, as well as to ensure that they acknowledge the underpinning theoretical considerations of their activities.

Health promotion in action

Part of the planning stage of McGhan et al.'s (2002) attempts to implement a whole schools based asthma management policy was to set up a committee to establish the issues surrounding asthma management, and then the viability of a health-promoting policy provision. The committee comprised a whole raft of different local community based services. This committee later became the steering group that facilitated communication between the key stakeholder groups.

Nurses should be cautious about using planning models if they are unfamiliar with their theoretical constructs, are new to health programme planning, or are merely looking for something to 'fall back on' if their interventions fail. On their own, planning models are no panacea for poor health education or health promotion practices; neither do they offer 'quick-fix' solutions. In the case of any planning process, and particularly those involving community development programmes, it can be two to three years before real progress is seen. Armed with this insight, nurses are far more likely to witness positive outcomes for their health promotion efforts.

Why do we need to plan health promotion?

It is clearly established that the more systematic, structured and well planned our health promotion activities are, the more likely they are to be both effective and successful (Tones and Tilford 2001; Green and Kreuter 2005). As with health promotion assessment, the more we plan effectively, the more we go in ready and prepared. Effective health promotion planning ensures that nurses identify and sign-post the necessary step-by-step stages and sequences for their health-related interventions. In turn, this ensures that they are provided with an overview of the main issues that require attention, that these issues are dealt with on a systematic basis, and that a checklist is at their disposal during the planning process

Health promotion planning is a 'dynamic process' (Pender et al. 2006): health promotion planning models help to prevent the development of ineffective health programmes and reduce any wasteful use of resources. They facilitate this by encouraging regular assessment of issues and progress throughout health promotion programmes. This aids situations in that nurses in the final stages of health interventions can identify where impact has occurred and how effective it has been. This requires more than a 'face value' measure. Some health professionals are known to struggle with planning processes. However, nurses are amongst those who are best suited to conduct it well, because a large part of nursing practice routinely plans for effective interventions for a range of client related health issues.

How do we plan health promotion?

To date, the nursing literature does not report on the utilization of the generic contemporary health promotion models – such as the Precede-Proceed model described earlier in this chapter. However, there are examples where health promotion models have been developed for specific health professional disciplines. This is particularly the case with nursing. Pender's Health Promotion model is the most used and tested planning model within nursing. It is a US based model (centred on a US-centric medical model of public health) that, while acknowledging wider social determinants of health, is noted more as a socio-cognitive behavioural model (Whitehead 2001a). Such a model is useful, but more suited to individualized health education interventions.

Whitehead's (2003a) Effect Planning Model for Health Promotion is representative of a health promotion model that has a community focus (see Figure 4.2). It is primarily designed for nurses, but the principles and activities can be applied to any health profession discipline. It is a model that places the nurse in different roles, working collaboratively with other disciplines and agencies, and mainly working as a health policy advocate and enabler. As a health promotion planning tool, the Effect Planning Model for Health Promotion allows nurses to see what types of activities are involved, what activities need to be monitored and what outcomes are desirable. It demonstrates that health promotion is a wide-reaching process that demands diverse skills of nurses.

Tones and Tilford's (1974) Planning Model for Health Education has been adapted and revised as a complex and linear effect model that is most likely to appeal to experienced health promoters. It differs from Green and Kreuter's Precede-Proceed Model in that it is primarily focused on educational outcomes.

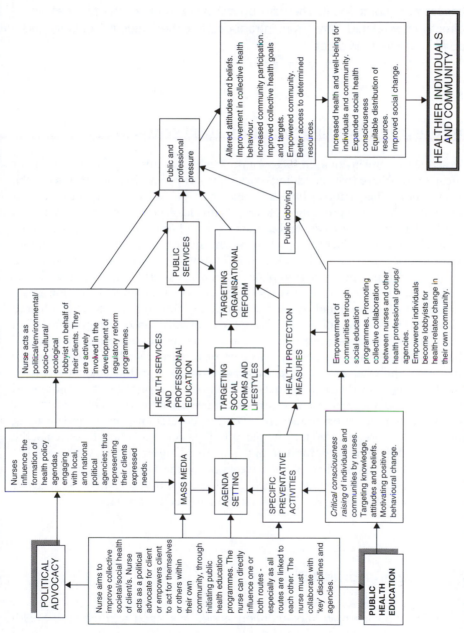

Figure 4.2 Whitehead's effect planning model for health promotion

Source: Whitehead (2003a).

> ### Summary point
>
> The planning phase of the health promotion process follows on from the assessment component. They are both integral parts of the process and directly inter-related. Any errors introduced in either stage will directly and adversely affect the other.

Implementing health promotion interventions

To describe the implementation stages of the health promotion process, you might be inclined to believe that the 'doing' part of health promotion would deserve the most attention. The paradox, though, is that there is less to write about here than other parts of the health promotion process. With clear and effective assessment and planning, the whys, wherefores and know-how of a health promotion programme is a natural follow-on. Where comprehensive and sustained assessment and planning have taken place, there is far less likelihood of anything untoward occurring and, hopefully, the health promotion implementation runs relatively smoothly (Tones and Tilford 2001). The main activities to remember in the implementation phase are that original assessed and planned activities and timeframes are being adhered to; due process is being followed; effective communication on progress between stakeholders is in evidence; and that any issues, barriers and dilemmas are reported and acted on accordingly. In effect, this part of the process adheres to a series of mini-reviews and evaluations (see *process evaluation* later in this chapter). It is by regularly performing this activity that nurses monitor progress, act on presented issues and change the course of any intervention where necessary. This is not to say that health promotion programmes are inflexible. Programmes might deviate along the way from the original plan for a whole raft of reasons but, where this occurs, the change must be deemed appropriate and be agreed between all key stakeholders (Whitehead et al. 2004). This is not a weakness of the health promotion process but, rather, an acknowledgement of its dynamic and fluid state. Nurses who favour frameworks that allow a degree of flexibility will appreciate this fact.

 Tutorial brief 4.5

Imagine that you are now implementing a well assessed and planned health promotion intervention. List the trouble-shooting measures that you might consider would assist the smooth running of the implementation stage.

Health promotion in action

Gomm et al. (2006) describe their community based public health advocacy campaign in Western Australia. A community alliance, concerned with heavy road traffic through a small regional city, negotiated solutions and identified two main targets for action. They implemented a range of initiatives that targeted a media advocacy strategy to attract public attention and reframe subsequent media messages. They also targeted policy alternatives to local government and industry standards. They were successful in putting pressure on key stakeholders in achieving their two main goals. This resulted in better public transport systems for shared use and the use of expanded rail services for freight transport for local industry.

Summary point

The 'doing part' or implementation of health promotion actually requires the least amount of 'processing'. If effective assessment and planning parts of the process have taken place, then implementation should run relatively smoothly. The focus in this part of the health promotion process lies mainly with ensuring that agreed due process is being followed, and that any necessary deviations are actively negotiated between key stakeholders.

Evaluating health promotion

With the evaluation stage of the overall process, health promotion programmes are able to establish whether their interventions have been effective, cost efficient and successful. As an essential activity in its own right, health promotion evaluation has a potential role at all stages of health programme provision. With this 'end point' to health promotion programming, nurses have a clear means of identifying whether the intervention has naturally completed or, as is the cyclic nature of health promotion, at what point one intervention ends and another starts. Subsequently, Naidoo and Wills (2000) have identified that evaluation is vital to ensure the ongoing survival and viability of health promotion.

Many nurses are under the impression that, if they plan their health promotion activities clearly, they will ultimately prove to be successful. This is true where effective planning also attends to the evaluation phase even before a programme of activities has begun. While effective assessment and planning are to be commended, on their own they are of limited value. Health promotion programmes require that all components of process are adhered to and this, therefore, must include a concerted evaluation phase. Evaluation is, perhaps, the most important part of any health promotion intervention. That said, of all the stages of health promotion process, the evaluation stage is the one least likely to be implemented. Many authors concur with this sentiment, and have remarked that the failure of many health promotion strategies – and the difficulty for them in being accepted into mainstream academic and clinical settings – is attributable to a lack of evaluative evidence (WHO 1998; Learmonth and Mackie 2000; Abbema et al. 2004). Positively, there are good nursing examples to draw upon that use evaluative process well (for example, Ashley et al. 2001; Twinn 2001; Lazenbatt et al. 2001; Bolman et al. 2002).

Additional point

Health promotion evaluation can be viewed as a research approach in its own right and, as such, involves assessing the capacity and performance of an intended intervention for health improvement, in terms of its effectiveness and efficiency.

Why do we need to evaluate health promotion?

Evaluation is an essential activity for any health promotion programme. The sometimes controversial and contested nature of what constitutes health promotion practice means that evidence of best practice and best outcomes needs to be provided. According to Naidoo and Wills (2000), health promotion can be an 'uncertain business', with no guarantees that the outcomes of programmes will deliver what is anticipated or required of them. Instead, attention to detail in the evaluative phase in most cases validates what has gone on previously, as well as provides real means with which to measure the position, validity, outcomes and success of health promotion programmes as they progress.

According to Downie et al. (1996), there are several reasons why we evaluate health promotion programmes – for instance, if nurses wish to assess the level and extent to which programmes have achieved and are achieving their objectives, as well as ensuring efficient and cost effective use of resources. Health promotion evaluation also informs the development of programme methodology, ensures that ethical and legal process is adhered to and helps to assess the place of health promotion activity in relation to its overall efforts to achieve health gain. Everitt and Hardiker (1997) identify two main reasons for wanting to evaluate health promotion activity. First, the need to generate hard evidence about the health promotion strategy being monitored and, second, the desire to make valued judgements on how good the interventions really are. Evaluation is therefore conducted for three overarching reasons: *future programme development, accountability* and *knowledge-building*. Another important advantage of evaluating health promotion programmes is that it allows nurses to design and implement new ones. This way nurses can learn from the strengths and weaknesses of previous programmes. Reviewing previous health promotion programmes becomes an integral part of health related work as nurses become more conversant with evaluative techniques. Kiger (1995) observes that those who evaluate their health promotion programmes also demonstrate their willingness to show accountability for their success or failure. Nurses who do this are demonstrating their willingness to be transparent and open.

How do we evaluate health promotion?

Health promotion evaluation can be a complex process because it asks a number of things of nurses. In the first instance, it requires that they choose an appropriate evaluation technique for the programme undertaken. Downie et al. (1996) identify the two 'main' types of evaluation for health promotion activity:

- *Outcome evaluation* This is evaluation that involves assessing an activity as a measure against specific aims or objectives. For instance, this might entail the overall impact of a one-year diabetes education programme. Essentially, outcome evaluation refers to the measurement of 'what has been achieved' – usually as the health promotion activities are drawing to a close – and necessitates that the researcher refer back to the original programme objectives. Outcome orientated evaluation is favoured where the objectives are evidence focused and effectiveness is an important aspect of the programme (Wimbush and Watson 2000).
- *Process evaluation* This approach is concerned with measuring an activity against a standard that might or might not be related to the specific objectives of the activity. This approach focuses more on 'how the intervention has been achieved', and tends to be measured as part of the programme process as it progresses. For instance, this might involve thinking about how well the different stakeholders collaborated together during the health promotion activity.

Process evaluation might not only consider the success rates of health promotion programmes, as outcome evaluation indicators tend to do, but also the processes of how success is achieved, how it is measured and at what cost. Outcome evaluation is, thus, primarily directed at resources and procedure related indicators.

Health promotion in action

Abbema et al. (2004), in a Netherlands-based community health project in a deprived area, demonstrate how they use *outcome mapping evaluation* (derived from an *intervention mapping* method) to identify programme objectives from which outcome measures could be derived. Although no significant health improvements in local residents were noted, the study showed that this type of evaluation could be used in a comprehensive community approach without compromising the processes of their health promotion interventions.

Indicator, process and outcome measures need to be known for the effective evaluation of health promotion. A wide range of health indicators exists, but they are mainly represented by *health profiles* (descriptive quantitative accounts of differing aspects of health) and *health indices* (the aggregating of different aspects of health performance into a single value). Difficulties in determining appropriate indicators for measuring success highlight the need for appropriate definitions of anticipated outcomes (Twinn, 2001). Perhaps the most commonly used *performance indicators* in health promotion are the three Es: *effectiveness, efficiency* and *efficacy*. Effectiveness is the extent to which a programme has met its intended objectives, efficiency is a measure of 'relative' success (in other words how successful the programme has been overall, even if it has not met all its intended objectives and outcomes) and efficacy is a measure used interchangeably between both effectiveness and efficiency (Tones 2000). As a measurement of the capacity of a programme to be accessed by all participants within a targeted community, the term *equity* can be added to the three Es.

 ## Tutorial brief 4.6

Imagine that you have implemented a community targeted health promotion programme. In terms of evaluation, identify the factors that would help you determine whether that programme had been successful?

Many nurses, when they do use evaluative methods, tend to choose singular techniques to monitor the processes of their health promotion activities. It is best practice to incorporate both process and outcome techniques when circumstances allow. A focus on *outcome evaluation* alone is known to limit the opportunity to learn valuable lessons about the approach itself (Downie et al. 1996). When combining a process and outcome approach in the same health promotion strategy, the evaluation then focuses on monitoring the process of change that occurs as the result of a health intervention, as well as monitoring the factors that facilitate or prevent desired changes. Britton et al. (1998) particularly recommend the use of quantitative outcome evaluation combined with qualitative process evaluation. Similarly, the WHO (1998) suggests that process evaluation, combined with short- and long-term outcomes, provides the best range of information for evaluating health promotion programmes.

Process and outcome evaluations are by far the most commonly utilized methods, but are by no means the only types of evaluation that can be used in health promotion programming. *Structural evaluation*, as it relates to the organizational and human resource influences on any health promotion programme, and *developmental, impact* and *transfer evaluation* processes are also worthy of mention (Kiger 1995). *Developmental evaluation* refers to assessment of the feasibility of a new programme and tests the effectiveness of a new approach. *Impact evaluation* is the assessment of the short-term immediate effect of a programme. *Transfer evaluation* is the assessment of 'replicability' (repeatability) of programme processes and outcomes, and their transferability to other settings or populations. A number of contemporary texts and sources elaborate further on these evaluation methods (for example, Schalock 2000; Oakley 2001).

Health promotion in action

Smith et al. (2004) report their Australian 'Eat Well SA Project', which aimed to increase consumption of healthy foods in children and their families. They used process and impact evaluation, as well as evaluated 'generative impact' (changes in organizational relationships). Using a capacity building framework, they identified that partnership development among key stakeholders and workers from child care, education, health, transport and food industry sectors met their intended outcomes. A model for planning and evaluating nutrition based health promotion emerged.

Hawley et al. (2007) describe their involvement in the aims of the public health Workforce and Leadership Development (WALD) Centre in Kansas, USA. This centre implements public health education and training projects through the collaborative processes of health needs identification, programme conceptualization, determining research initiatives and health promotion programme evaluations. They put forward several case studies to promote the success of project outcomes, using this partnership formula.

Although some nurses might view health promotion evaluation as a somewhat complex process, even the modest methods of evaluation can be used routinely in practice (Ewles and Simnett 2003). Whitehead's (2003b) evaluation model (see Figure 4.3) is an example of a simplified stage process model that represents a mostly linear sequence of events to be addressed in order to ensure that health promotion evaluation is as effective as possible. All evaluation sequences, however, must be cyclical if they are to succeed, because this facilitates the re-defining and setting of new goals, as well as the reformulation of any unmet outcomes. This is highlighted in Whitehead's model. The early stages of this model are aimed at identifying the process and purpose of the evaluation strategy. Following on from these stages are the logistical and resource implications of conducting evaluation research. Nurses are guided by the model through a comprehensive planning phase that eventually leads to the implementation and final evaluation of the programme. Success is often measured in terms of the outcomes met, although this does not mean that not meeting the intended outcomes equates to an unsuccessful programme. For example, the programme might not meet original objectives but, instead, uncover newer and more appropriate objectives to be pursued in another or a continuing project. Therefore, outcomes might change or success might be measured in terms of lessons learned. Alternatively, the meeting of all intended outcomes might equate to a completed programme that is then terminated.

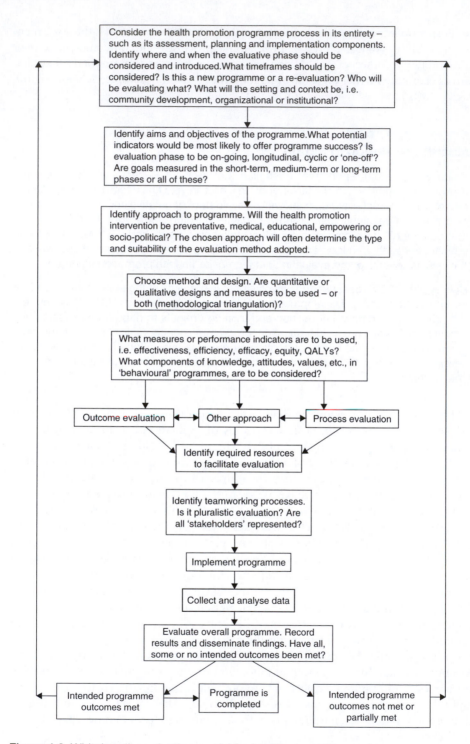

Figure 4.3 Whitehead's evaluation model for health promotion
Source: Whitehead (2003b).

A systematic process for health education

So far, in this chapter, we have explored the systematic and structured processes of health promotion. As discussed in Chapter 1, health education can be a very useful adjunct to or sub-set of health promotion. However, health education on its own, while likely to be part of an overall broad health promotion strategy, is viewed as a far more limited health approach than health promotion (Casey 2007; Irvine 2007). This is particularly so when engaging in socio-cognitive related behavioural change activities (see Chapter 2). Whitehead (2001a) has developed a nursing-specific socio-cognitive model (see Figure 4.4). Pender's Health Promotion model, really a health education model (see Figure 2.5), is a good example of a nursing-specific socio-cognitive behavioural model.

It is well known that nurses have been, and continue to be, heavily reliant on traditional forms of socio-cognitive and behavioural-orientated health education. This type of health education, in isolation, is usually an activity that facilitates the professional assessment of an individual's health status against causal risk factors associated with lifestyle related behaviour. Following this assessment, if health risk (preventative approach) or actual ill health/disability (medical approach) is determined, nurses strive to educate, and subsequently motivate, the individual (in a group context or otherwise) to engage in a behavioural change process as a means for the prevention of, or the stabilization of or improvement in, a negative health status. Behavioural change, however, in any individual, is both extremely complex and fraught with dilemmas for health educators. The intention in this section of the chapter is not to criticize this form of health intervention. If health education activity, in both its limited and more expansive forms, is currently the mainstay of nursing health-related practice, what is most important to identify is the extent to which less limited forms can be promoted and a higher level of successful outcome predicted. Subsequently, as outlined in Chapter 1, it can be determined which health education programmes better link and engage with the wider processes of health promotion.

Whitehead and Russell (2004) confirm that traditional health education activity represents the majority of current health professions health-related activity. They are not critical of this fact but, instead, put forward recommendations for ensuring that such practices are as encompassing and wide-reaching as possible. This is both to aid better client related outcomes and to align such activities to health promotion process.

In summary, they recommend the following activities when conducting health education interventions:

- Considering whether the behavioural change intervention is appropriate and realistic in the first place
- Making clear to the client the nature and intent of the intervening health education activity
- Factor for client 'resistance' and 'reactance' behaviours
- Present health information in an unbiased manner, not as a 'moral good'
- Not to filter or censure health information
- Consider health information in the context of 'health protection'
- Explore client's health related beliefs, values and attitudes

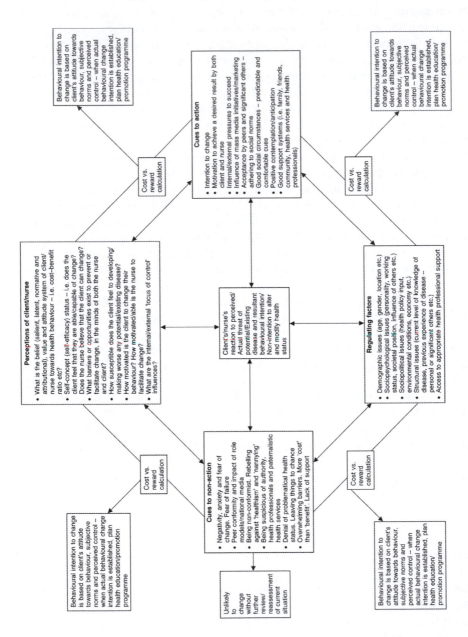

Figure 4.4 Whitehead's socio-cognitive model for health education

Source: Whitehead (2003a).

- Be aware that clients' personal assessment of health status might be distorted
- Accurately assess past behavioural history
- Assess emotional capacity for behavioural change – ensure the client is not too anxious or stressed
- Negotiate behavioural priority on the basis of clients' priorities
- Assess the health beliefs and influence of significant family members
- Assess impact of client's socio-environmental situation
- Ensure that the health education programme is well planned, resourced and evaluated
- Ensure that health education programme has realistic and achievable aims and objectives
- Ensure that health education programme combines information-giving and behavioural adaptation alongside social 'skills-building' activity
- Ensure that health education programme utilizes a wide range of designs and methods
- If at least some of the above-mentioned processes are not possible, it is *best* to avoid implementing them in the first place

Accommodating as many of these listed activities as possible, as well as underpinning them with an identifiable socio-cognitive behavioural model, will increase the chance of successful health education programme outcomes. At the same time, especially if planned and implemented well, these outcomes will fit well with wider health promotion activities and outcomes.

Health promotion and the process of research

This section complements some of the content in Chapter 6 but, here, focuses on research as an integral part of an underpinning overall process of health promotion. As well as needing to know current evidence bases for a health promotion programme prior to its implementation, it is also necessary to determine the most suitable research method to adopt. Until quite recently, a positivist approach to health promotion programmes has predominated. The traditionally viewed 'optimum' research design in the field of medicine has been the *randomized controlled trial* (RCT). With the historical influence of medicine on health care, this research design has been predictably applied to a significant proportion of health promotion research. More recently, this situation has been strongly challenged by those in the field (Learmonth and Watson 1999; Ashley et al. 2001). Indeed, even the WHO (1998: 6) argues that the use of RCTs in most cases is an 'inappropriate, misleading and unnecessarily expensive' method of researching health promotion. This is not just the case with RCTs, but can also apply to other experimental research methods. The ideological underpinning of health promotion activity has never really lent itself well to the deconstructionist leanings of impersonal research frameworks. Personal health experience is seen to be an essential component of health promotion activity, where it is ideologically unsound to reduce people to mere objects in health promotion research (Raphael and Bryant 2000). Wass (2000) states that community action and policy change activity is not actually amenable to pure quantitative analysis methods. Instead, in the case of community action strategies, participatory styles of research are seen to be far more appropriate (see *action research* later in this chapter). Peersman et al. (1999) identify that, currently, health professionals are beginning to look beyond traditional and dominant research paradigms to adopt the most appropriate methodology for the task at hand while synthesising the best aspects of available research tools.

What nurses should guard against, when it comes to choosing the most appropriate method(s) for researching health promotion, is rejecting any approach 'out-of-hand', or merely choosing whatever method is in vogue at the time. It has become evident that no single research approach is appropriate for all situations. There are many methods to choose from, and the health professional is advised to seek out those that are most relevant to the aims and needs of their chosen programme activity. Rolls (1999) argues that health promotion activities need to be based on their own terms and not underpinned by different criteria and values. Instead, it is wiser to adopt a *realistic evaluation* approach which is not simply driven by method or measurement, neither should it be performed solely for the benefit of science but, rather, driven by practitioners for the benefit of the programme participants and the public (Pawson and Tilley 1997). Flexible modes of incorporating both quantitative and qualitative evaluative methods are now being recognized as a sensible way forward. Oakley (2001: 28) puts it well:

> What is important is that we leave behind the killing fields of the paradigm war and enter the more humane and kinder territory of combining methods and approaches in order to answer focused questions about how health promotion initiatives can enhance the quality and quantity of people's lives.

Health promotion in action

Hawley et al. (2006) utilize both quantitative and qualitative measurement in their rural setting childhood and adolescent obesity prevention health promotion programme. A specifically developed Health and Wellness questionnaire survey was used, which aimed, in the first place, to unearth a qualitative demographic and assessment of perception of community activities in addressing youth nutrition and exercise. The second part of the survey quantitatively uncovered data on psychological and cognitive skills, levels of physical exercise and nutrition states, behavioural attributes and skills, and the social, cultural and physical environment. Further on, local 'focus group' meetings and individual interviews took place, and a revised qualitative questionnaire was submitted.

Action research

In Chapter 6, participatory research is discussed and action research is briefly mentioned. This section elaborates action research further. Appropriate and wide-reaching methods are needed for conducting and evaluating health promotion research. Particularly, the use of action research is now advocated and encouraged by many health professionals (Whitehead et al. 2004; Saaranen et al. 2005; Liu et al. 2006). Koch and Kralik (2006: 121) state:

> Participatory action research methods are now increasingly used in the development of community health organizational partnerships. These projects put participation, action research and adult education at the forefront of attempts to liberate and emancipate disempowered people. Participatory action research methods are being used not only so that local people can inform outsiders, but also for people's own analysis of their own situation and conditions ... To the wider body of development programmes, projects and initiatives, participatory action approaches represent a significant departure from historical and standard practices.

Action research, in particular, engages both researchers and participants in processes that help to create collective empowerment, organizational change, community capacity-building, and meaningful action towards achieving equitable communities. These are modern and desirable outcomes for health promotion programmes today. In line with the earlier section on evaluation process, Tones and Tilford (2001) particularly stress the use of action research in *process evaluation*. Furthermore, as well as action research coming under the umbrella of participatory research, it is also a design that uses a *mixed method* approach (Whitehead and Elliott 2007). As discussed earlier in this section, mixed methods approaches encourage the use of both quantitative and qualitative data, as well as advocating for varied use of data collection and analysis processes. Figure 4.5 demonstrates the participatory change cycle for organizational change. The situation presented applies equally to both organizational or community change issues.

Additional point

There are many similar terms to describe different versions of action research – such as 'participatory action research', 'participatory research', 'participatory evaluation', 'developmental action research', 'action inquiry', 'mutual inquiry', 'action science', 'action learning' and 'empowerment evaluation'.

Health promotion in action

Liu et al. (2006) adopt a participatory action research (PAR) approach with their health promotion programme working with disadvantaged elders in the Shaanxi Province of China. PAR training was initially received from HelpAge International, followed by a two-year project that built up local sustainability through cooperation among all stakeholders and engendered the mobilization of local government. Focus group discussions with villagers and family visits provided the means to gather data. From this, workshops for local government officers and local elders evolved. Continuous evaluation sustained the overall programme.

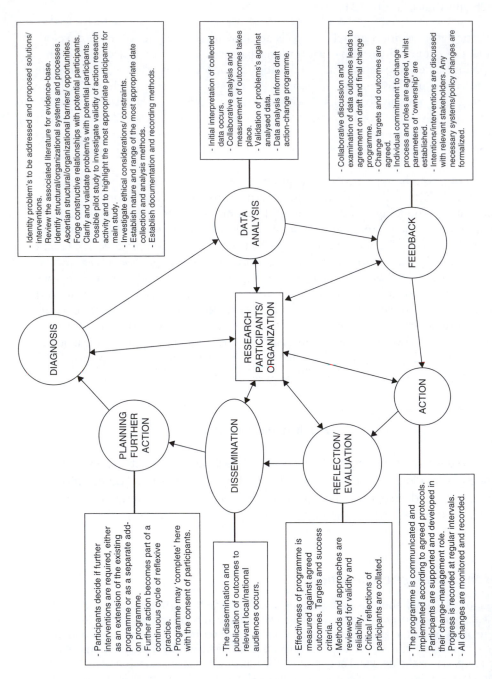

Figure 4.5 Whitehead et al.'s action research model
Source: Whitehead et al. (2003).

Health promotion and the process of evidence based practice

The systematic and structured processes already mentioned do not occur on their own without some form of evidence base to underpin them (see Chapter 6). It would be an unwise endeavour to attempt accurate assessment and the planning of a health promotion intervention in the absence of identifying and understanding the existing evidence base for the type of programme being contemplated. The same is so for the evaluative stages. It would make little sense not to compare and contrast the findings of 'completed' health promotion programmes with what has gone on before. Examining the current evidence base affords the health promoter the privilege of knowing what has previously occurred, and where the strengths of and gaps in similar interventions lay. Health promotion is clearly more effective when comprehensive approaches are based on sound evidence and are adopted accordingly (Scriven 2005).

The current global economic climate, accompanied by recent radical quality-related reforms, has led to an increased interest in monitoring health promotion initiatives (South and Tilford 2000; Learmonth 2000). Accessible and well-evaluated forms of evidence have become an integral part of health promotion practice. Raphael (2000) and Bartholomew et al. (2001) highlight the timely emergence of an increasingly high profile for health promotion and its evaluation, given the heightened presence of evidence based practice issues. How health professionals access evidence, and what that evidence base is, however, has been the source of fierce debate. The nature of the debate is twofold. First, it occurs where evidence based practice is aligned purely against performance management and cost saving exercises that are not usually priorities of health promotion. Second, debate occurs where the evidence base is directed purely by bio-scientific and positivist frameworks (South and Tilford 2000; Lazenbatt et al. 2001). These frameworks, alone, are not consistent with the underpinning philosophy of health promotion activity. There is a growing unease about the use of restrictive biomedically focused models of health in health promotion, and scepticism about the benefit of their health interventions, especially in relation to what is counted as a 'successful' health intervention (Browne 2001). Tones (2000), for instance, states that epidemiological indicators should *never* be used to assess health promotion programmes, while Downie et al. (1996) highlight the limitation of observing a disease orientated health state as the baseline, then measuring deviations from this, as a focus on ill health rather than positive health measurement.

While it is contested that rigid alignment to positivist experimental evidence might not be the best practice for health promotion, there is also a viable argument that it is prudent to base our practices on the 'best' available evidence. In fact, it might be considered negligent not to do so where good quality evidence is available that matches intended health promotion outcomes. For many, that will mean adhering to established hierarchies of evidence where the considered top standards are met by the systematic reviews of mainly randomized controlled trials and observational studies – such as with the Cochrane Collaboration (www.cochrane.org), the Cochrane Health Promotion and Public Health Field (www.vichealth.vic.gov.au/cochrane)

and the NHS Centre for Reviews and Dissemination (www.york.ac.uk/inst/crd/wph.htm) (see Chapter 6 for further detail). While this information, however, is available for some health promotion fields, it is still a resource that is yet to become available to many other fields of inquiry. This leaves a problem for many health promoters. Rychetnik and Wise (2004: 254–5) sum up this dilemma by stating:

> The greatest challenge for those who advocate evidence-based health promotion probably exists when they identify important health promotion goals (for example, based on evidence of need) for which the evidence to support intervention is either unavailable or inadequate ... there might be value in considering whether it is feasible to generate evidence, or whether the available evidence is the best that can be expected ... Such an analysis can assist advocates of evidence-based practice to weigh whether to lobby for better research or whether to pursue their policy and practice goals despite the limited evidence available.

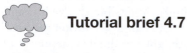

Tutorial brief 4.7

In the absence of 'quality' evidence, what other forms of evidence might you be able to access to assist with health promotion interventions?

Summary point

The need to satisfy demands that health promotion interventions adhere to the conventions of evidence based practice and also appropriate research methods (particularly participatory designs) means that these ventures must be considered against the overall context of the systematic process of health promotion.

Conclusion

Health promotion interventions should adhere to a logical, sequential and systematic process. In this chapter, the case has been put forward that – with good, sound and comprehensive attention to overall process – nursing related health promotion programmes are far more likely to be successful and to result in desirable and effective outcomes. Health promotion is a dynamic process that does not happen by chance. Knowing what the overall process is, and which parts and stages comprise that process and how they can be applied, significantly aids the nurse in conducting effective health interventions. Part of the overall process – not covered in this chapter, but extensively covered in Chapter 5 – is the understanding of the appropriate locations and settings for these processes to occur.

Additional resources

Hodges, B.C. and Videto, D.M. (2005) *Assessment and Planning in Health Programs* (Boston, MA: Jones & Bartlett).

Kreuter, M.W., Lezin, N., Kreuter, M. and Green, L.W. (2003) *Community Health Promotion Ideas That Work*, 2nd edn (Boston, MA: Jones & Bartlett).

Ottoson, J.M., and Green, L.W. (2001) 'Public Health Education and Health Promotion', in Novick, L.F. and Mays, G.P. (eds), *Public Health Administration: Principles for Population-based Management* (Gaithersburg, MD: Aspen): 300–23.

Society of Health Education and Promotion Specialists (2007) SHEPS – Practice, Principles and Philosophy, SHEPS. Available online at http://www.hj-web.co.uk/sheps/vision.htm (accessed 12 September 2008).

References

Abbema, E.A., van Assema, P., Kok, G.J., de Leeuw, E. and de Vries, N.K. (2004) 'Effect Evaluation of a Comprehensive Community Intervention aimed at reducing Socioeconomic Health Inequalities in the Netherlands', *Health Promotion International*, 19: 141–56.

Aponte, J. and Nickitas, D.M. (2007) 'Community as Client: Reaching an Underserved Urban Community and Meeting Unmet Primary Health Care Needs', *Journal of Community Health Nursing*, 24: 177–90.

Ashley, A., Lloyd, A., Lamb, S. and Bartlett, H. (2001) 'Is Health-related Quality of Life a Suitable Outcome Measure for Evaluating Health Promotion Programmes?', *Nursing Times Research*, 6: 671–8.

Bartholomew, L., Parcel, G., Kok, G. and Gottlieb, N. (2001) *Intervention Mapping: Designing Theory and Evidence-based Health Promotion* (Mountain View, CA: Mayfield).

Beattie, A. (1991) 'Knowledge and Control in Health Promotion: A Test Case for Social Policy and Social Theory', in Gabe, J., Calnan, M. and Bury, M. (eds), *The Sociology of the Health Service* (London: Routledge).

Berentson-Shaw, J. and Price, K. (2007) 'Facilitating Effective Health Promotion Practice in a Public Health Unit: Lessons from the Field', *Australian and New Zealand Journal of Public Health*, 31: 81–6.

Bolman, C., de Vries, H. and van Breukelen, G. (2002) 'Evaluation of a Nurse-Managed Minimal-contact Smoking Cessation Intervention for Cardiac Inpatients', *Health Education Research*, 17: 99–116.

Britton, A., Thorogood, M., Coombes, Y. and Lewando-Hundt, G. 'Letter – Search for Evidence of Effective Health Promotion', *BMJ*, 316: 703.

Browne, J. (2001) 'Commentary – The Limitations and Usefulness of Quality of Life Assessment in Healthcare', *Nursing Times Research*, 6: 679–81.

Caplan, R. and Holland, R. (1990) 'Rethinking Health Education Theory', *Health Education Journal*, 49(1): 10–12.

Casey, D. (2007) 'Nurses' Perceptions, Understanding and Experiences of Health Promotion', *Journal of Clinical Nursing*, 16: 1039–49.

Chiang, L.C. (2003) 'Educational Diagnosis of Self-management Behaviours of Parents with Asthmatic Children by Triangulation based on the PRECEDE-PROCEED model in Taiwan', *Patient Education and Counseling*, 49: 19–25.

Downie, R.S., Tannahill, C. and Tannahill, A. (1996) *Health Promotion: Models and Values*, 2nd edn (Oxford: Oxford University Press).

Everitt, A. and Hardiker, P. (1999) 'Towards a Critical Approach to Evaluation', in Sidell, M., Jones, L., Katz, J. and Peberdy, A. (eds), *Debates and Dilemmas in Promoting Health: A Reader* (London: Macmillan): 200–6.

Ewles, L. and Simnett, I. (2003) *Promoting Health: A Practical Guide*, 5th edn (London: Ballière Tindall).

French, J. and Adams, L. (1986) 'From Analysis to Synthesis', *Health Education Journal*, 45(2): 71–4.

Gandelman, A.A., DeSantis, L.M. and Rietmeijer, C.A. (2006) 'Assessing Community Needs and Agency – An Integral Part of Implementing Effective Evidence-based Interventions', *Aids Education and Prevention*, 18: 32–43.

Gomm, M., Lincoln, P., Pikora, T. and Giles-Corti, B. (2006) 'Planning and Implementing a Community-based Public Health Advocacy Campaign: A Transport Case Study from Australia', *Health Promotion International*, 21: 284–92.

Green, L.W. (1980) *Health Education Planning: A Diagnostic Approach* (Palo Alto, CA: Mayfield).

Green, L.W. (2005) 'Prospects and Possible Pitfalls of a Preventative Polypill: Confessions of a Health Promotion Convert', *European Journal of Clinical Nutrition*, 59 (supp1ement): 54–9.

Green, L.W. and Kreuter, M.W. (1991) *Health Promotion Planning: An Educational and Environmental Approach*, 2nd edn (Palo Alto, CA: Mayfield).

Green, L.W. and Kreuter, M.W. (1992) 'CDC's Planned Approach to Community Health as an Application of PRECEDE and an Inspiration for PROCEED', *Journal of Health Education*, 23: 140–7.

Green, L.W. and Kreuter, M.W. (1999) *Health Promotion Planning: An Educational and Ecological Approach*, 3rd edn (Palo Alto, CA: Mayfield).

Green, L.W. and Kreuter, M.W. (2005) *Health Program Planning: An Educational and Ecological Approach*, 4th edn (New York: McGraw-Hill Higher Education).

Hawley, S.R., Beckman, H. and Bishop, T. (2006) 'Development of an Obesity Prevention and Management Program for Children and Adolescents in a Rural Setting', *Journal of Community Health Nursing*, 23: 69–80.

Hawley, S.R., Molgaard, C.A., Ablah, E., Orr, S.A., Oler-Manske, J.E. and St Romain, T. (2007) 'Academic-practice Partnership for Community Health Workforce Development', *Journal of Community Health Nursing*, 24: 155–65.

Irvine, F. (2007) 'Examining the Correspondence of Theoretical and Real Interpretations of Health Promotion', *Journal of Clinical Nursing*, 16: 593–602.

Jackson, L. (2007) 'Health and Health Promotion', in Wills, J. (ed.), *Promoting Health: Vital Notes for Nurses* (Oxford: Blackwell): 11–27.

Kiger, A.M. (1995) *Teaching for Health*, 2nd edn (Edinburgh: Churchill Livingstone).

Koch, T. and Kralik, D. (2006) *Participatory Action Research in Health Care* (Oxford: Blackwell Publishing).

Kreuter, M., De Rosa, C., Howze, E. and Baldwin, G. (2004) 'Understanding Wicked Problems: A Key to Advancing Environmental Health Promotion', *Health Education & Behavior*, 31(4): 441–54.

Lazenbatt, A., Orr, J. and O'Neill, E. (2001) 'Inequalities in Health: Evaluation and Effectiveness in Practice', *International Journal of Nursing Practice*, 7: 383–91.

Learmonth, A.M. (2000) 'Utilising Research in Practice and Generating Evidence from Practice', *Health Education Research*, 15: 742–56.

Learmonth, A. and Mackie, P. (2000) 'Evaluating Effectiveness in Health Promotion: A Case of Re-inventing the Millstone?', *Health Education Journal*, 59: 267–80.

Learmonth, A. and Watson, N. (1999) 'Constructing Evidence Based Health Promotion: Perspectives from the Field', *Critical Public Health*, 19: 317–33.

Linnan, L.A., Sterba, K.R., Lee, A.M., Bontempi, J.B., Yang, J. and Crump, C. (2005) 'Planning and the Professional Preparation of Health Educators: Implications for Teaching, Research and Practice', *Health Promoting Practice*, 6: 308–19.

Liu, M., Gao, R. and Pusari, N. (2006) 'Using Participatory Action Research to Provide Health Promotion for Disadvantaged Elders in Shaanxi Province, China', *Public Health Nursing*, 23: 332–8.

MacDonald, T.H. (1998) *Rethinking Health Promotion: A Global Approach* (London: Routledge).

McGhan, S.L., Reutter, L.I., Hessel, P.A., Melvin, D. and Wilson, D.R. (2002) 'Developing a School Asthma Policy', *Public Health Nursing*, 19: 112–23.

McMurray, A. (2007) *Community Health and Wellness: A Socio-ecological Approach*, 3rd edn (Marrickville, Sydney, Australia: Elsevier/Mosby).

Naidoo, J. and Wills, J. (2000) *Health Promotion: Foundations for Practice*, 2nd edn (London: Baillière Tindall).

Nuñez, D.E., Armbruster, C., Phillips, W.T and Gale, B.J. (2003) 'Community-based Senior Health Promotion Program using a Collaborative Practice Model: The Escalante Health Partnerships', *Public Health Nursing*, 20: 25–32.

Nutbeam, D. and Wise, M. (2004) 'Structures and Strategies for Public Health Intervention', in Detels, R., McEwan, J., Beaglehole, R. and Tanaka, H. (eds), *Oxford Textbook of Public Health* (Oxford: Oxford University Press): 1873–88.

Oakley, A. (2001) 'Evaluating Health Promotion: Methodological Diversity', in *Using Research for Effective Health Promotion*, Oliver, S. and Peersman, G. (eds) (Buckingham: Open University Press): 16–31.

Pawson, R. and Tilley, N. (1997) *Realistic Evaluation* (London: Sage).

Pender, N.J., Murdaugh, C.L., and Parsons, M.A. (2006) 'Health Promotion in Nursing Practice, 5th edn (Upper Saddle River, NJ: Pearson/Prentice Hall.

Peterson, D. and Alexander, G.R. (2001) *Needs Assessment in Public Health: A Practical Guide for Students and Professionals* (New York: Kluwer Academic).

Peersman, G., Oakley, A. and Oliver, S. (1999) 'Evidence-based Health Promotion?. Some Methodological Challenges', *Journal of the Institute of Health Education*, 37(2): 59–64.

Raphael, D. (2000) 'The Question of Evidence in Health Promotion', *Health Promotion International*, 15: 355–67.

Raphael, D. and Bryant, T. (2000) 'Putting the Population into Population Health', *Canadian Journal of Public Health*, 91: 9–12.

Rolls, L. (1999) 'The Challenge of Evidence-based Practice', in Perkins, E.R., Simnett, I. and Wright, L. (eds), *Evidence-based Health Promotion* (Chichester: John Wiley): 47–50.

Rychetnik, L. and Wise, M. (2004) 'Advocating Evidence-based Health Promotion: Reflections and A Way Forward', *Health Promotion International*, 19: 247–57.

Saaranen, T., Tossavainen, K. and Turunen, H. (2005) 'School Staff Members' and Occupational Health Nurses' Evaluation of the Promotion of Occupational Well-being – With Good Planning to Better Practice', *Journal of Interprofessional Care*, 19: 465–79.

Savelson, A., van Wynsberghe, R., Frankish, J. and Folz, H. (2005) 'Application of a Health Promotion Model to Community-based Sustainability Planning', *Local Environment*, 10: 629–47.

Schalock, R.L. (2000) *Outcome-based Evaluation* (London: Kluwer Academic).

Scriven, A. (2005) 'Promoting Health: A Global Context and Rationale', in Scriven, A. and Garman, S. (eds), *Promoting Health: Global Perspectives* (Basingstoke: Palgrave MacMillan): 1–13.

Smith, A., Coveney, J., Carter, P., Jolley, G. and Laris, P. (2004) 'The Eat Well SA Project: An Evaluation-based Case Study in Building Capacity for Promoting Healthy Eating, *Health Promotion International*, 19: 327–34.

South, J. and Tilford, S. (2000) 'Perceptions of Research and Evaluation in Health Promotion Practice and Influences on Activity', *Health Education Research*, 15: 729–41.

Thomson, P. (1998) 'Application of the Planning Compass to the Nursing Curriculum: A Tool for Health Promotion Practice', *Nurse Education Today*, 18: 406–12.

Tones, K. (2000) 'Evaluating Health Promotion: A Tale of Three Errors', *Patient Education and Counselling*, 39: 227–36.

Tones, K., and Tilford, S. (2001) *Health Promotion: Effectiveness, Efficiency and Equity*, 3rd edn (London: Nelson Thornes).

Twinn, S. (2001) 'The Evaluation of the Effectiveness of Health Education Interventions in Clinical Practice: A Continuing Methodological Challenge', *Journal of Advanced Nursing*, 34: 230–7.

Wass, A. (2000) *Promoting Health: The Primary Health Care Approach*, 2nd edn (Sydney, Australia: Harcourt).

Whitehead, D. (2000) 'Using Mass Media within Health-promoting Practice: A Nursing Perspective', *Journal of Advanced Nursing*, 32: 807–16.

Whitehead, D. (2001a) 'A Social-cognitive Model for Health Promotion/Health Education Practice', *Journal of Advanced Nursing*, 36: 417–25.

Whitehead, D. (2001b) 'A Stage Planning Process Model for Health Promotion/Health Education Practice', *Journal of Advanced Nursing*, 36: 311–20.

Whitehead, D. (2003a) 'Incorporating Socio-political Health Promotion Activities in Nursing Practice', *Journal of Clinical Nursing*, 12: 668–77.

Whitehead, D. (2003b) 'Evaluating Health Promotion: A Model for Nursing Practice', *Journal of Advanced Nursing*, 41: 490–98.

Whitehead, D. and Elliott, D. (2007) 'An Overview of Research Theory and Process', in Schneider, Z., Whitehead, D., Elliott, D., LoBiondo-Wood, G. and Haber, J. (eds), *Nursing and Midwifery Research: Methods and Appraisal for Evidence-Based Practice*, 3rd edn (Marrickville, Sydney, Australia: Elsevier/ Mosby): 20–32.

Whitehead, D., Taket, A. and Smith, P. (2003) 'Action Research in Health Promotion', *Health Education Journal*, 61: 5–22.

Whitehead, D., Keast, J., Montgomery, V. and Hayman, S. (2004) 'A Preventative Health Education Programme for Osteoporosis', *Journal of Advanced Nursing*, 47: 15–24.

Whitehead, D. and Russell, G. (2004) 'How Effective are Health Education Programmes: Resistance, Reactance, Rationality and Risk? Recommendations for Effective Practice', *International Journal of Nursing Studies*, 41: 163–72.

WHO (1998) *Health Promotion Evaluation: Recommendations to Policymakers*, Report of the WHO European Working Group on Health Promotion (Copenhagen: WHO).

Wimbush, E. and Watson, J. (2000) 'An Evaluation Framework for Health Promotion: Theory, Quality and Effectiveness', *Evaluation*, 6: 310–21.

Wills, J. (2007) 'The Role of the Nurse in Promoting Health', in Wills J. (ed.), *Promoting Health: Vital Notes for Nurses* (Oxford: Blackwell): 1–10.

Wise, M. and Signal, L. (2000) 'Health Promotion Development in Australia and New Zealand', *Health Promotion International*, 15: 237–48.

CHAPTER 5

Settings Based Health Promotion

Dean Whitehead

Objectives

By the end of this chapter you should be able to:

- Identify the concept and frameworks of the health-promoting settings movement
- Explore how different settings are related to each other
- Examine how different settings impact on health promotion practice
- Identify existing limitations of current settings based roles and functions
- Establish where the nurse's role and function exists or could be implemented in working within identified settings

---

Key terms

- Community development
- Health promotion
- Health-promoting health services
- Health-promoting hospitals – HPHs
- Health-promoting schools – HPSs
- Health-promoting workplaces – HPWs
- World Health Organization – WHO

Introduction

In the mid-1980s, the World Health Organizations' (WHO) *Ottawa Charter for Health Promotion* paved the way towards the development of a series of 'settings based' health promotion strategies, where specific health related settings were designated for special attention (WHO 1986). The Ottawa Charter supported certain settings being nominated as unique social systems for enabling specific health promotion activity. These settings initially included community, schools, workplace, and the home and family. A number of other settings have since been added to the list, now including health-promoting universities (HPUs) (Xiangyang et al. 2003; Whitehead 2004a) and health-promoting prisons (HPPs) (Watson et al. 2004; Whitehead 2006a). Other authors have hinted at the possibility of establishing other unique settings – such as health-promoting general practices, nursing homes, and churches (Wass 2000; Peterson et al. 2002; Watson 2008).

This chapter chooses the most relevant main settings for nurses working in health services, and explores their function and place. For this chapter, that means identifying the issues surrounding health-promoting health services generally – and, more specifically, hospitals, schools and universities. Health-promoting prisons are purposely excluded, as only a relatively small group of nurses work in correctional care. For those who are especially interested in this setting, though, several nursing articles cover nursing related health promotion issues associated with prison services (Watson et al. 2004; Whitehead 2006a). The initial focus of this chapter lies with the current predominant settings for nurses working in the health services; namely, the hospital or clinical institution. Reading through this whole chapter, though, the reader should note that it is the community setting that encapsulates and is central to all the settings combined.

Why settings for health promotion?

As already stated in the introduction, the high profile development of the settings-based approach to health promotion continues to be actively reinforced by the WHO. Weare (2002) states that the settings based approach to health promotion remains the 'big idea' of the WHO's vision of health promotion. Hesman (2007) identifies that health promotion always takes place in 'settings', where settings are environments in which people learn, work, play and love – and that these settings have profoundly influenced health promotion approaches. Both Weare (2002) and Dooris (2005) emphasize that a settings approach to health promotion is focused on the 'total context' in which health related activity occurs. This is where the surrounding environment, ethos and relationships either support or undermine health. Dooris and Thompson (2001) note the settings role of advocating for the active development of healthy public policy at the local and national level. As with all health promotion activity, the settings based role is politically motivated and orientated. Supporting this, many institutions within health settings are either government or state controlled.

Later settings based reform has steered away from a traditional emphasis on just physical and environmental surroundings as they impact on the health of individuals, and has moved towards an approach where action visibly takes place at the socio-ecological level. For nurses and all health professionals, settings define and locate health structures within organizational contexts and parameters. The capacity and extent to which settings and their organizational structure have adapted and worked towards broader social health reform is an indicator of effective health promotion process and outcome (Poland et al. 2000).

While there are clear differences between the identified settings, it is important to remember that there are obvious overlaps as well. For instance, it is difficult to separate out health-promoting schools and universities completely since, although they might deal with differently aged clients, their activities and outcomes are still centred on education and health as a lifelong process. It is easier, however, to separate out prisons and schools, for example – but there still remains a relationship between the two settings. For instance, they come together when nurses have a role in young offenders centres.

It is clear that the outcomes for health promotion strategies, in any setting, will ultimately be the same; that is, addressing the issues that directly and indirectly affect the health status of those contained within and served by the setting. The intention is that, although these settings exist as distinct entities in their own right, they are also supposed to be 'seamlessly' intertwined within the community in which they are contained and which they serve. In terms of broad health promotion strategies, one setting will almost invariably impact on another. Evidence suggests that this is particularly so for nursing (Whitehead 2005). This is most apparent in the noted links between health services that serve both the hospital and community settings. In an ideal world, all designated settings would lay within the broad remit of community. Aligned to this context, community is where *all* people work and dwell (Hesman 2007).

Health promoting health services

The section following this one deals with health promoting hospitals. For the majority of nurses reading this chapter, the hospital is where their primary practice will be based. That said, authors have expanded this narrower focus to explore the wider concept of health promoting health services – or a 'whole systems' approach (Dooris et al. 2007). This will obviously incorporate traditional acute based hospital services, but also wider based community examples as well. For instance, some authors have identified the concept of health promoting general practices (Starfield 2001; Watson 2008). While community based, such practice establishments (also incorporating community outpatient clinics, drop-in centres and health centres) are closely linked with acute services, and tend to be run and structured on similar medical models of care.

Health promotion in the hospital setting

The health promoting hospital (HPH) movement began in Europe in 1998, having been preceded by a range of WHO-centred legislative and guideline based documentation. This included *The Budapest Declaration on Health Promoting Hospitals* and *The Vienna Recommendations on Health Promoting Hospitals* (WHO 1991, 1997). Since then, there have been attempts to bring about further settings based health promotion expansion and reform in hospitals. As institutions with the potential to engage in active promotion of the health and well-being of its users and workforce, hospitals have consistently been targeted by many countries as the first settings based 'port of call'. Some countries have been particularly keen to enforce a concerted mobilization of the HPH concept into their institutional settings. In the UK, for instance, government driven legislative documentation has explicitly recognized the potential of health-promoting hospitals (DoH 1994, 2004). Such legislation has had a profound impact on the way that nurses practise in the hospital setting, with drivers for reform centred more on social functions of health rather than pure biotechnical drivers. Hospital based nurses, who note that their practices are based more on the processes of social models of health as opposed to biomedical models of health, are in the best position to appreciate the wider dimensions of a health-promoting hospital approach.

The HPH movement has enjoyed, and continues to enjoy, a steady expansion of its network, although it is difficult to gauge its exact momentum and impact. Groene (2005) indicates that there are now 25 member states with 35 national and regional European HPH Networks that, since January 2001, have seen the number of signed-up health-promoting hospitals rise from 534 to more than 700. These figures however, only represent the position in Europe. It is difficult to assess the world-wide impact of the HPH movement because the WHO does not offer specific figures in relation to its global position. Johnson (2000) offers a global estimate (by now, dated) suggesting that there are about 1000 hospitals included in the global HPH network, spanning 32 countries. These figures, when compared with Groene's figures, suggest that the vast majority of HPH related activity occurs within the European community.

What does a health-promoting hospital do?

The noted hesitancy of many hospitals to embrace health promotion strategies often lies with the lack of clarity over what an HPH is and does. Many hospitals have subsequently sought to embrace the concepts according to their own interpretations, but usually with mixed results. To help overcome this, the WHO (1997), in its document *The Vienna Recommendations for Health Promoting Hospitals*, drew up a recommended framework as a general guideline for activities that would make a hospital health-promoting. They are expressed as:

- A holistic focus on health activities and interventions that improve the clients' overall well-being – as opposed to biomedically orientated and disease based curative services that focus only on physical health
- The prioritization and subsequent resourcing of services contributing to enabling and empowering patient-focused interventions
- Encouraging participation that is action focused, egalitarian and equal for users according to their health potential
- Fostering organizational commitment through encouraging participatory, health gain orientated procedures that involve all professional groups, and foster alliances with professionals outside the hospital setting
- Expanding the hospital's public health role, in alliance with the population of the local community and its social and health services, therefore optimizing links

between different providers, users and actors in the 'whole' health and social care sector
- An investment in training and educating health personnel and lay activists, as well as developing leaders and specialists, in areas relevant to hospital based health promotion strategies.

This list represents an ambitious aim for any hospital or collection of hospitals to achieve, but it is recognized that aiming to establish at least parts of the framework would benefit nurses and their clients. In other words, effective partial reform would have better outcomes than over-ambitious and ineffective total reform.

In accordance with some of these listed recommendations, Pelikan et al. (1997) identify that an HPH engages several activities at the same time. First, it uses episodes of acute injury or illness as an opportunity to promote health through providing and organizing rehabilitation.

Second, it encourages, liaises with and empowers clients to make better use of primary health care services. Third, and most importantly, it acts as an agent for health development of the whole community – through networking with local health related services in order to build alliances for continuous care and health promotion.

When reviewing the noted recommendations, a repeating pattern emerges. Most visible is the organizational obligation to meet the changing and evolving health care needs of the local community. As part of recently emerging reform programmes throughout the world, many hospitals are required to demonstrate a notable shift from a focus on acute based curative service functions towards delivery of health services across the whole health and social care continuum. The HPH movement, as an adjunct to this reform, incorporates the principles of capacity-building and organizational change as part of a concerted re-orientation of service delivery that promotes health within and outside its physical boundaries. What has become clear is that the HPH movement represents one of the main drivers for a more holistic partnership approach to health service delivery. Johnson and Baum (2001) state that, until a hospital is truly a health promoting organization in its own right, it cannot broaden its approach to improve the health of the community that it serves. Therefore, a broader vision sees the development of not merely what could be termed as health-promoting hospitals but, rather, institutions that could be termed 'public health hospitals'. These hospitals develop their staff to move away from a focus on medicalized sub-specialization to an increasing understanding of the wider health agenda (Wright et al. 2002).

 Tutorial brief 5.1

Do you work, or have you worked, in a hospital based setting that promotes the principles of a health-promoting hospital? If so, what activities have you observed, and how do they impact on client and health professional services? Could more be done in your identified organization? If so, what?

Additional point

Not all hospitals that actively pursue health promotion strategies will be recognized under the WHO's HPH standards. Ironically, some hospitals that are registered as HPHs might have achieved this barely meeting minimal standards. The poorer a country is in terms of its overall health service infrastructure, understandably, the more likely that this will be the case.

Box 5.1   The qualities of a health-promoting hospital

- Ensuring that clients and staff are enabled to achieve their maximum potential for a positive health and well-being status – raising awareness
- Developing a commitment within the institution to implement 'wholesale' organisational reform – based on a health promotion rationale
- Multi-professional/agency collaboration in health-related research and clinical practice
- Appropriate representation of all relevant parties – particularly lay public and client representation
- Creating supportive and empowering health-promoting environments for practitioners and clients alike
- Commitment to effectively train and educate all health professionals on matters of health promotion
- Developing hospital-based health policies to reflect health promotion outcomes
- Developing integrated and 'seamless' links between the hospital and surrounding community setting
- Working towards a gradual 'demedicalization' of services. Here, the practitioner does not instinctively adhere to a negative health, disease-orientated regime of treatment but, instead, considers why the client is presenting with their condition and what can be done to foster well-being while they are in hospital and beyond.

The impact and limitations of health promotion in the hospital setting

While the progress of the HPH movement has been steady, it has not constituted a universal shift to date. As early as 1989, Lalonde commented that hospitals were not heeding the call to incorporate health promotion activity into practice, suggesting that often hospitals felt that some other setting would do it instead (Lalonde 1989).

Weil and Harmata (2002) state that, because of their need to focus on fiscal management issues, many hospitals have set aside their mission to promote and protect the health of surrounding communities. More recent commentary continues in this vein, noting that most hospitals are still hesitant about incorporating health-promoting principles into their structure, organization and culture (Bakx et al. 2001; WHO 2003). There are many reasons why this is the case, although most can be pinned down to traditional organizational structures and processes. For instance, Guilmette et al. (2001) state that the hospital demands of reducing in-patient stay periods and other functional outcomes ensures that, often, health promotion issues do not receive due attention. Subsequently, it is known that the complex organizational structures of many hospitals serve to exclude many of its health professionals from exposure to broad health promotion activities. Where this occurs, nurses are unable to associate health promotion as a valid part of their role or function (Casey 2007; Irvine 2007). Authors refer to the lack of progress made and the need for further health promotion reform in hospitals, as they trail behind other health and social care settings in their attempts to incorporate health promotion initiatives into their service role (Johnson and Baum 2001; Rustler 2002).

The HPH movement is based on the assumption that health promotion improvement is the most effective vehicle for organizational development. That having been said, much of its activity could currently be more appropriately defined within the context of health educating hospitals. The available literature mainly describes disease management objectives and outcomes, with a particular focus on the target of promoting 'smoke free' hospitals (Quinn et al. 2001). Such limited targets, however, do not sit well with the broader aims of health promotion and the HPH movement. Where these types of 'health education' programmes are in place, they are often further limited by the fact that they occur as isolated projects in relation to the rest of the organization.

Positive ways that nurses can contribute to the health-promoting hospital movement

Johnson (2000) reports that the increasing interest in matters of disease prevention and health promotion has led to a growing awareness of the limitations of acute medicine. She adds that hospital administrators are also now beginning to recognize that a hospital's reputation and image, in line with patients' growing expectations, needs to be based on positive health based outcomes, not ill health and emergency treatment. A greater emphasis on positive health and well-being, in place of a negative emphasis on ill health, is part of proposed HPH reforms. For many nurses, health promotion can only be effectively incorporated into the health services alongside an agenda of gradual demedicalization and the further enhancement of personal control for clients' health (Goel and McIsaac 2000). If it is to be realistic and representative, health promotion should acknowledge the social, economic and environmental contexts of health, as well as the biological. This promotes a realization that health-promoting hospitals are focused on issues wider than introducing a variety of information-giving techniques as a means for changing health behaviour. However, where these activities are used, there needs to be recognition that cognitive behavioural change programmes involve extremely complex multi-variant behavioural processes (Whitehead and Russell 2004). However, it is argued that comparatively little effort is required from health institutions in order to make the transition from health educating to health promoting hospitals. This perception is captured by the words of Johnson and Baum (2001: 281) who state:

> So although hospitals are the high temples of sick care, the extensive resources that they command means that even a small shift of focus has the potential to bring about an increase in resources dedicated to health promotion and, in time, health benefits to the community

Health promotion in action

Põlluste et al. (2007) describe their Estonian based HPH study of both registered and non-registered HPH institutions. An extensive survey of 54 Estonian hospitals was based on the WHO quality assurance standards for developing HPHs. The study showed that those hospitals that were HPH registered with the WHO were far more likely to adopt whole organization practices based on linking quality assurance to health promotion activities. They noted better health services, well-being and health of patients and staff in the hospitals that could demonstrate high quality assurance standards. Shifts to incorporate quality assurance programmes were proven not to be too demanding or resource intensive. Guo et al. (2007) have conducted a similar study between managers in Beijing based hospitals in China.

At least limited health promotion reform must be undertaken if hospitals are to avoid existing in 'splendid isolation' from the overall health of the communities that they serve (Wright et al. 2002). Encouragingly, even if the examples are still a little scant, some authors report the developing of hospital based health promotion outreach programmes that describe a concerted partnership between them and the surrounding community (Mavor 2001; Quinn et al. 2001).

From the position of nurses themselves, there is recognition of the need to move beyond any reluctance to carry out a health promotion role within the hospital setting (Chan and Wong 2000). Where nurses have a positive belief in health promotion, this is mirrored in their subsequent commitment to facilitating health promotion programmes. Where this occurs, much of the success has been attributed to all health professionals convincing hospital based dignitaries that health promotion initiatives ease, rather than add, any organizational reform burden, as well as improve chances for overall effectiveness and provide fresh ways to tackle existing problems (Pelikan et al. 2001). This activity involves recognition that consumers of hospital based health care – our clients – are more discerning and informed on matters regarding their health than ever before. They are fast becoming a powerful lobby that is beginning to demand a say and choice in determining their own regimes of care. Many nurses recognize this as a fundamental right for their clients. This sentiment has long been endorsed by the WHO (WHO 1988 cited in Hartrick et al. 1994: 86), who state that:

Health-improving activities must go further than merely providing professional service to passive recipients. Rather, health promotion includes concrete public participation where people are active agents and decision makers, as opposed to consumers of a service provided by health professionals.

As well as collaborating with clients, it is important to acknowledge the importance of multi-professional and multi-agency collaborative practice in hospitals. This does not merely involve the traditional collaborations within the organization (doctors, allied health professions (AHPs) and nurses), but also the less established collaborations such as with managers/administrators, service personnel, clients and lay activists. Significantly, it has to include similar collaborations with the representatives of community based health service organizations, local businesses, voluntary and charitable organizations, political organizations and local community action groups. These representatives make up the types of key stakeholder that must be present for health promotion programmes to be effective.

Instead of dealing with health promotion issues that are limited to localized ward/unit based practices, the HPH movement offers nurses the scope to address factors that pertain to 'whole system' organizational change and community related public health issues. Within this lies an acknowledgement that hospitals exists as a whole organization or system, and that each ward, unit or service facility represents only a component of that structure. Individual wards and units can initially serve as the focus for broader organizational reform through focusing on the 'health-promoting ward'. Coakley (1998) argues that focusing on health promotion in the ward setting can facilitate a wider public health role for nurses, but only if the 'peripheral services' that are often associated with them are acknowledged. Recent developments are helping to facilitate this. I refer to the increasing amount of nursing related literature that describes the notions of the 'hospital in the home' (Duke and Street 2003) and 'home healthcare' (Thome et al. 2003). Nurses in hospitals could look to this growing movement as a direct link to the community, whereby staff could move freely between the acute and community setting and share expertise.

Health promotion in action

Bensberg et al. (2003) describe their study that explored ways of making an emergency department (ED) more health-promoting for nurses and other health professionals. They conducted workshops with community representatives – such as local councils, community health services, general practices, police, health monitoring and data collection agencies, state government health departments and non-government specialist health promotion groups – to see how their ED services could be improved. Successful outcomes meant that all parties were willing to collaborate with the ED to improve immunization strategies and diabetes services, initiate appropriate referrals for drug and alcohol abuse programmes, identify comprehensive discharge planning strategies, tackle inappropriate referrals to the ED and forge better links overall with community-based services.

Summary point

Hospitals are one of the more difficult environments into which to introduce HPH programmes. These acute based institutions are more typically based on medicalized and curative treatment based functions and regimes that do not sit well with health promotion activities. Despite being situated in the 'heart' of communities, paradoxically, hospitals often isolate themselves from existing community health services. This having been said, it is known that this situation is improving and that it only requires quite small shifts in position to promote radical health promotion reform for nursing and nurses.

Health promotion in the school setting

Many nursing related groups (including midwifery and health visiting services) have links with schools, even if these links are not always obvious. This might be through paediatric, maternal or social services. Other specific groups – such as school nurses, health visitors and specialist community public health nurses – will have more obvious involvement. The fact is that preventative health promotion strategies often dictate that nurses intervene in the early stages of the life span continuum in seeking to instil healthy practices that younger people will take with them into their middle-adult lives and beyond. The school setting is seen as one of the most important health related growth and 'front-line' defence areas for health promotion and health education intervention, where health promotion policies are a vital and integrated part of national curricula and health services (Tossavainen et al. 2004). From this position the health-promoting school (HPS) movement has emerged.

What does a health-promoting school do?

Although the HPS concept was one of the first to emerge from the *Ottawa Charter*, its formal conception was quite slow in the making. It was not until 1995 that an expert WHO commissioned committee proposed a set of HPS related guidelines, demonstrating six component areas, which were identified as:

- The physical environment of the school
- Health policy of the school
- The social environment of the school
- Community relationships (inclusive of links to parents, families and outside agencies)
- Personal health skills
- Relationship with health services (WHO 1995a).

From these broad guidelines, the HPS is meant to demonstrate how it achieves a healthy environment for its total population, through developing supportive health promotion structures. In effect, they are supposed to demonstrate a move away from the traditional school structures that cling on to the culture of a dominant academic function, hierarchy and limited autonomy for all (Scriven and Stiddard 2003). In response to the HPS concept, we have witnessed a concerted effort to move away from 'inappropriate' classroom-based/individualized disease prevention health education approaches towards much broader structures and processes (Deschesnes et al. 2003).

The HPS strategy has also marked a concerted attempt to move on from traditional health related school programmes and curricula, where health-promoting related interventions have mainly followed a preventative lifestyle and behaviour focused health education route. This is particularly the case because emerging evaluative results for such programmes of delivery have identified very little impact on the health attitudes and behaviours of the school population (Schofield et al. 2003). The HPS movement now acknowledges that it is better for schools to aim to be educational settings that are capable of a concerted capacity for healthy learning, living and working through the taught curriculum. Schools are therefore more likely to evidence explicit health-promoting processes through the adoption of those demonstrated in the frameworks and concepts of *eco-holistic models* and conceptual well-being modes (Konu and Rimpela 2002).

A growing number of authors refer to the fact that progressive and sustained health promotion schools related reform is based on the principles of empowerment, democracy, partnership, equity, action competence, social capital and sustainability (Jensen et al. 2000). These are principles that are echoed in the mandate of the HPS movement, but are not exclusive to it. Many school institutions are now able to demonstrate that their students, school staff, parents and health agencies are driven by a health-promoting policy process that encourages participation, self-determination, citizenship and agency.

 Tutorial brief 5.2

List the positive and negative factors of the school setting for implementing and promoting health promotion.

The impact and limitations of health promotion in the school setting

A great deal of investment, in terms of human and structural resources, is needed for sustained health promotion activity in the schools environment. In recognition of this, the implementation of HPS strategies is not without its dilemmas, and subsequently is 'rarely' implemented as intended (Deschesnes et al. 2003; Scriven and Stiddard 2003). Even though the WHO (2008) describes the school setting as an 'extraordinarily effective setting in which to improve people's health', nurses need to be aware that it is also one of the most problematic areas for health promotion activities. Various reviews of HPS study evaluations have concluded that targeted 'whole school' implementation of health promotion strategies has often not been realized where the intention was to do so (Curless and Burns 2003; Estabrooks et al. 2003). The 'closest' examples that can be found to a collaborative whole school and surrounding community health promotion capacity and process are presented in the findings of certain authors (Larsson and Zaluha 2003; Eliason and True 2004; Berg et al. 2004). It is interesting and positive to note that these examples are all nursing led.

Additional point

It is important to note that, while schools represent a huge potential to initiate health promotion principles, they are not always the most positive environments for children to learn these principles. Negative experiences, such as bullying and peer responsiveness, might stand in the way of health promotion activities.

Another problem for the HPS movement lies in the evidence surrounding the role and working position of those whose services are employed to implement schools based health promotion reform – often including nurses. The nursing based literature often cites a lack of appropriate training and preparation, a lack of research evidence and evaluated health programmes, confusion about role, and the discipline not being appropriately recognized, valued or resourced by managers and other health professional colleagues (Larsson and Zaluha 2003; Barnes et al. 2004; Croghan et al. 2004; Whitehead 2006b). Furthermore, Bagnall (1997) has suggested that health professionals often find themselves in a 'rut', caught between the divisions of both health and educations services, and consequently failing to find a place within the overall primary health care team. This has not been good for the morale, confidence or position of representative nursing groups. Such factors have led to a rapid turnover of nursing staff and a feeling of a lack of defined career progression, meaning that many are leaving such services and not being replaced (Croghan et al. 2004).

Health promotion in action

Sun and Stewart (2007) report on their research to investigate the relationship between a health-promoting schools (HPS) approach and social capital. Social capital is characterized as a resource that resides in the relationships between people and key health stakeholders and what resources can be drawn upon to achieve positive socially related health actions. Their findings suggested that there is a significant relationship between HPS indicators and social capital. They go on to argue that an HPS approach to build social capital in schools is an effective framework for health professionals to adopt.

Positive ways that nurses can contribute to the health-promoting schools movement

Studies have identified that, in order for nurses working directly within school settings to move their health promotion/public health position forward, they must develop a coherent and collective health strategy alongside a body of good quality outcome based research evidence to measure this activity (Wainwright et al. 2000; Bartley 2004). Together with this, it is suggested that nurses must also ally themselves to specific health promotional and educational outcomes (Maughan 2003). Another important development is that all health professionals identify themselves as one partner in an overall collaborative health schools effort. DeBell and Everett (1998) identified their Healthy Schools Award Scheme as one example of incorporating a multi-agency health professions resource, with school nursing leading the way. McGhan et al. (2002) also report their successful school asthma policy programme, which includes the collaborative efforts of key stakeholders such as community nurses, pupils, parents, school staff, health educators, paediatricians and environmental health specialists. Meanwhile, Tossavainen et al. (2004) highlight cross-discipline efforts to include parents, school staff, and social and municipal services – such as youth workers. This mirrors other authors' assertions that, to reflect true multi-sectoral cooperation, effective HPS programmes require partnership between all education, health professional and social service agents (Lee et al. 2001; Deschesnes et al. 2003). Also of interest is Plews et al.'s (2000) observation from their study that nurses working in acute hospital trusts were developing links to school related health activities. Hospital based health professionals are just as capable and well placed as community based colleagues to develop school based interventions. It would represent a milestone in the health-promoting settings movement if they were seen to be aligning the activities of health-promoting hospitals (HPHs) with those of an HPS framework (Whitehead 2004b).

Health promotion in action

Mäenpää et al. (2007) report their school nurse led health project involving Finnish sixth-graders. Twenty-two sixth-graders (aged 11–12 years) became participants in their grounded theory study. Their findings suggested that pupils thrived and their health benefited where individual counselling and coping skills were reinforced alongside informative interaction with the family unit.

Summary point

The school is one of the more important health promotion settings for a number of reasons – but mainly because instilling positive health promotion activity in younger children has the potential to change the health status of whole communities over a period of time. Although fraught with dilemmas that might not occur in an adult based population, investment in this setting is seen as a priority for the WHO and nursing.

Health promotion in the university setting

In line with the fact that universities are aiming for increasing numbers of students yet financial support for most students is decreasing, universities have to take more responsibility for acting as 'supportive environments for health'. Stock et al. (2001) report that university students identify with a strong need for personal access to health promotion facilities, especially in relation to psychosocial stress counselling and alcohol abuse strategies. Universities are realizing that they need to invest in health programmes that are inherently embedded within the culture and systems of their organizations for the benefit of students, staff and the wider community.

Throughout the Western world there are examples of concerted efforts to set up health-promoting university (HPU) networks, but reform is still in its infancy. For instance, the American Network of Health Promoting Universities (ANHPU) has approximately 72 institutional members, through its links with the Association of Academic Health Centres (AHCs). Hampshire (2003: 4) reports that several influential United Kingdom organizations – for example, the Health Development Agency, the Healthy Settings Development Unit, Universities UK, the National Union of Students and the Department of Health – have set up an HPU planning group, going on to state that:

> Potentially, this could lead to a national framework for health-promoting universities that would cover everything from the quality of buildings and environment to management styles, as well as policies on sexual and mental health and drinks and drugs misuse.

What does a health-promoting university do?

An HPU aims to provide similar services to all other health-promoting settings in providing a wide range of health promotion and health education initiatives. Tsouros et al. (1998: 3) state that an HPU should broadly seek to:

- Protect the health and well-being of students, staff and the wider community through effective and innovative policies and practices
- Increasingly direct its teaching and research capacity towards health promotion activities
- Develop concerted health promotion alliances and outreach facilities with its surrounding community

An HPU seeks to serve the needs of its immediate student and staff population. At an individual level, university based health promotion programmes offer the potential not only to affect the health related behaviours and lifestyles of health professionals that access them, but the opportunity for nurses and other health professionals employed on the programmes to have direct access to the student and staff population. Health promotion initiatives in the university setting are particularly useful because not only does the health promoter have the capacity to reach a potentially captive audience, but also the opportunity to instil healthy practices in the young adults who make up the majority of the student population might result in a lifetime of positive health related activities. Studies have already demonstrated how important it is to target students' health related knowledge and beliefs as a means of instilling early and sustained healthy behaviour (Xiangyang et al. 2003). Hampshire (2003) reports on a health education initiative that has targeted a popular nightclub venue for university students and employed volunteers to hand out 'goody bags' containing safer sex and drug use information, along with condoms and novelty stickers. Palmer (2003) also puts into practice the notion of deploying health promotion specialists to develop educational programmes that could assist the organization and its employees in dealing with work related stress.

Naturally, with a high young adult student population, the available examples currently identify priority areas for such programmes and interventions that include mental health, occupational health and safety, sexual health, illicit drug and alcohol consumption, nutritional health, food safety, physical exercise, design and transport facilities, and building structure (Petkeviciene et al. 2002). These issues, however, are not exclusive to the student population and might also target university based staff, including nurse educators.

The impact and limitations of health promotion in the university setting

Settings based health promotion strategies require that nurses work outside conventional spheres of practice, and often outside the health service domain. The university is such a place where health services can have a huge impact. In North America, the ANHPU states that it is particularly 'eager' for the involvement and the development of Schools of Public Health at participating higher education institutions. Reger et al. (2002), however, highlight the fact that, while universities might be rich in health related resources, they are often limited by a disease focused orientation. The involvement and influence of medically orientated health faculties and programmes in universities might compound this dilemma.

Positive ways that nurses can contribute to the health-promoting universities movement

Beyond the boundaries of the actual institution, the most important thing that an HPU can acknowledge is that it is a community resourced, driven, and serving facility – not a self-serving organization that exists in isolation of its neighbouring community. Subsequently, recent calls have encouraged academic–community partnerships as a means of addressing particular community driven public health issues (Levy et al. 2003; Whitehead 2004a). A forward thinking university will seek to initiate collaborative research forums at senior levels in order to fulfil health-promoting objectives that will be considered of value to the local community. It is recognized that 'authentic' university–community participation is difficult to achieve, but examples do exist where this has happened (Maurana et al. 1998; Levy et al. 2003). From examples such as these, the links to potential community funding and working with partnership organizations are clear. Geiger et al. (2002) particularly stress the opportunities that are presented through health promotion partnerships between public schools and universities. Dooris (2001) states that universities, through their own policy processes, have the capacity to build health into other organizations through 'contract specification'. In particular, he goes on to argue that the expertise and influence of a university means that it can develop an advocacy role that will influence healthy public policy at local, national and international levels.

Health promotion in action

Xiangyang et al. (2003) report their health-promoting setting study in a Beijing University, which took place over a one-year period. They focused on health policy issues for creating a healthy physical and social environment, a reorientation of offered campus health services and interventions for developing student and staff personal health skills. After a year, evaluation showed that 75 per cent of students and 83 per cent of staff reported a significant increase in physical and social environmental facilities. A third of students reported an increased mental health capacity, and increased numbers reported positive changes in lifestyle behaviours.

Those nurses who are seeking to develop a specialist clinical or academic health promotion/public health role through accessing university-based degree awards are a particularly valuable and potentially influential resource for any university to tap into. Universities could be viewed as testing grounds, where the theoretical and practical components of health education and health promotion modules and programmes serve as a valuable starting or continuity point for clinical practice. In essence, the university could be seen as not only a good breeding ground for nurses to learn broad health policy and health promotion skills, but also a useful location for disseminating these skills to both a localized and wider audience. This helps to establish the location of professional and personal health promotion practice within a wider social and political context.

Health promotion in action

Huyhn et al. (2000), as part of a university-based teaching-learning community clinical practicum programme, report how nursing students helped to set up a health information Internet site within an under-served inner city high school. It allowed students to experience at first hand the sustainable practices of community orientated participation. Local solutions to community health problems were uncovered and credibly linked to the university sector. It is acknowledged that the local community provides students with the opportunity for health related discovery and development, while adding to the validity of service learning from an academic perspective (Maurana et al. 1998).

> ### Summary point
>
> A university is a useful setting for developing health promotion programmes. It is closely linked to the HPS setting as part of lifelong learning skills for younger adults – but it is also the setting where many nurses will train and further develop their skills.

Health promotion in the workplace

The health-promoting workplace (HPW) is fast gaining pace as one of the more important health promotion settings (Shain and Kramer 2004). It holds a unique place, in that the health and wellbeing of workers inevitably impacts on the health of individual families, the local community and society at large. Its boundaries therefore extend and cross over into the domains of other settings. The European Region WHO website is dedicated to the HPW concept, and details over 300 related publications that are linked to the strategy (WHO 2008).

What does a health-promoting workplace do?

According to the WHO (2008), a comprehensive workplace health promotion scheme empowers social partners from both inside and outside workplace enterprises for the health maintenance of workers and their families, and creates healthy working environments for them. The WHO adds that those who implement such schemes must have a good working knowledge of health factors as they relate to lifestyle, structural, occupational, environmental, ecological and social determinants of health within and outside of organizations.

 Tutorial brief 5.3

1. What are the positive and negative factors of health related activities in your place of work that affect both your health and work related practices?

2. How could the negative factors that you have identified be addressed?

In their most desirable form, HPW initiatives take on the shape of an organizational capacity-building approach. Authors have identified what properties such health-promoting capacity-building processes require (Germann and Wilson 2004;

Whitehead 2006c). These authors point out that organizational capacity-building is associated with a range of strategies that include:

- The building up of infrastructure to address organizational health and social issues
- Firmly embedding health promotion programmes in organizations
- Sustainability of health promotion schemes after initial phases
- The health related problem solving capacity of organizations as it relates to individual members and their surrounding community
- The integration of health promotion knowledge across organizations and communities for the long term
- Integrated organizational support for associated policies and procedures
- A genuine commitment to the processes that foster health promotion capacity

The impact and limitations of health promotion in the workplace setting

Organizational policies that address workplace health and lifestyle issues can be powerful indicators of an organization's commitment to employee health and welfare. It is well established that a healthy workforce affords the employer far more benefits. For instance, investing in workplace health schemes provides organizations with motivated workforces, higher morale, reduced absenteeism, reduced personnel and welfare problems, reduced industrial relationship disputes, increased overall efficiency and improved organizational performance, competitiveness and public image (Chu et al. 2000). The consequences for any organization that has an unhealthy workforce are many and include work related accidents, high rates of absenteeism, high levels of stress, loss of productivity and high incidence of health related litigation (Verow and Hargreaves, 2000; Johnson et al. 2003). Interestingly, Kessler et al. (2004) identify the phenomena of 'presenteeism' as a direct result of ill health amongst employees. This is where employees present at work but provide inadequate work performance. Ironically, health care professionals (with nurses rating highly) have the highest rate of 'sickness presence' or presenteeism when compared with other sections of industry (Aronsson et al. 2000).

Additional point

Carlson and Warne (2007) have identified that there is a direct link between the health status and working health of nurses and their ability to conduct health promotion. They advocate 'action learning' as a means to help nurses link their positive personal health status to implementing health promotion in practice.

It is reported that many health service employers continue to do little to address broader determinants of health within an organizational capacity. They prefer, instead, to focus on the priorities of immediate acute care services (Germann and Wilson 2004). The conventional activity associated with the HPW movement, so far, has mainly centred on physical and psychological behavioural lifestyle-related objectives and outcomes – such as smoking and alcohol/illicit drug-monitoring, stress reduction, mental health schemes, employee fitness and exercise, weight control, prevention, early detection and screening programmes for serious diseases, back care, healthy eating, health information programmes and health paraphernalia (Holdsworth et al. 2004; Cleary and Walter 2005). The WHO related documentation on workplace health promotion to date also tends to centre on occupational health factors, although this looks set to change. In 1995, the WHO released its *Global Strategy on Occupational Health for All: The Way to Health at Work* recommendation report (WHO 1995a), espousing, in principle, the right of all workers to health at work and a healthy working environment. Behaviourally orientated workplace health schemes tend to have, at best, 'modest' outcomes (Holdsworth et al. 2004). In essence, health programmes that focus merely on personal lifestyle factors, at the expense of not addressing structural and environmental organizational issues, are somewhat limited. Current healthy workplace schemes, therefore, have to look more broadly than behavioural change frameworks if they are to achieve sustainable reorientation of health-promoting health services.

Positive ways that nurses can contribute to the health-promoting workplace movement

When referring to healthy workplaces, many nurses might think purely in terms of the workplace and employee situation as it relates directly to the confines of their immediate institutions – such as hospitals or health centres. Many nurses, however, work outside these traditional organizations – such as in industry, business or social services. While the perception of traditional organizations is understandable, it is argued that nursing managers should also be aware that healthy workplaces provide the added benefit of access to large numbers of individuals who are also part of the wider social community. Ennals (2002) reminds us that we are obliged to consider the world beyond the workplace – the one in which nurses are engaged as citizens. Subsequently, and in line with the public health commitments of health service organizations, the extension of a positive healthy culture in the workplace is the potential influence on the health of immediate and wider family groups of health employees. Community health action is also useful for encouraging healthy lifestyles in the workplace as part of a social normalization process. It is wise to consider the image that health services project into the communities that they serve, not only through the health standards and status of their patient outcomes, but also through the health status of their local workforces. With the mention of patients, however, it would also be remiss not to consider the further health contribution that HPWs have on those for whom health services are designed – the clients. Kearsey (2003) has already highlighted that healthy workplaces also equate to healthier patients.

Additional point

It is important to note that health-promoting workplaces do not only relate to the traditional institutions in which nurses work – particularly the hospital setting. While issues of the HPH movement impact on the workplace, this is only one setting within which nurses work, and where healthy workforces make a significant and positive health impact on services and clients. Many nurses work outside traditional structures and organizations – such as in industry, business or social services, where workplace health promotion issues are equally as relevant.

Health promotion in action

Guo et al. (2007), in their study, identify the direct link between knowledge of health promotion in hospital based managers and their willingness to promote health in the workplace. Where managers had a clear understanding of the potential and actual impact of health promotion, the health of workers and clients was far more likely to experience positive health outcomes. Where these were daily practices, it was identified that this was accompanied by a managerial commitment to providing appropriate personnel, funding and training.

An organizational base line assessment or audit will initially be required, if new healthy workplace schemes are to be adopted. The first step in improving workplace health is to realize what is needed and what is acceptable, and to move beyond the situation whereby organizations have lost touch with the fact that environments need to change. Germann and Wilson (2004) argue that, primarily, organizations need to address the 'inward evaluative gaze', whereby workplaces engage with people to build capacity for creating healthier environments and communities. The WHO stresses that health outcomes are best considered in relation to evaluation at the community level, especially using work related and public health indicators (WHO 2008). As such, aligning business objectives with public health initiatives is a key element in developing effective workplace health promotion activities.

Health promotion in action

Runciman et al. (2006) report on their health promotion related study into work practices of community nurse with older people. The survey revealed that, where effective and creative group work at the inter-disciplinary, multi-disciplinary and multi-agency levels, then effective health promotion activity was in evidence in the workplace. The barriers to effective health promotion in the workplace with regard to older people existed where there was a lack of planning (especially involving clients), audit and evaluation, and where there was a lack of funds.

In order to move away from the limitations of conventional healthy workplace strategies, current sustainable workplace health interventions require that nurses address a number of different issues to ensure success. Wilkinson et al. (1997) suggest that this broader focus needs to lie with organizational development, human resource management, training, marketing, communication, multi-disciplinary collaboration, and multi-method evaluation. Supportive interpersonal relationships at work, workplace culture, training and support to learn jobs, and effective approaches to staff management are key to the success of workplace health promotion. As Ennals (2002: 45) states:

> It is time for 'joined up thinking' across disciplines and departments, involving the development of partnership relationships, including social partnerships. This is not an alternative to financial investment, but a means of transforming workplace relationships so that investments can be more effective. It means continuing conversations and increasing the responsibilities of the work of workplace health and hygiene professionals in a changing world.

Summary point

The workplace is where nurses spend a great deal of their lives. How workplaces are structured and organized has a strong influence on our health and practices, as well as the health of our clients. The better the work environment, the more likely it is that health promotion activities will be in place.

Conclusion

If health-promoting settings are to move beyond the situation where they exist as 'an idealism that sounds good in theory' for nurses and nursing (Cullen 2002), a concerted review of health promotion activities by the nurses who work in those settings is due. It makes sense to view our health promotion practices, not just in the context of individual projects in individual settings, but in terms of whole organizational or whole community impact and outcomes. Thinking beyond the scope of the immediate practice or setting to consider the links between, and influences of, other settings has enormous positive health benefits for those that work in them and access their services. Current evidence, in most settings, suggests that concerted and universal health promotion reform is still to be realized in nursing, but is being worked towards.

Additional resources

Dooris, M. (2004) 'Joining Up Settings for Health: A Valuable Investment for Strategic Partnership', *Critical Public Health*, 14: 37–49.

Groene, O. and Jorgensen, S.J. (2005) 'Health Promotion in Hospitals – A Strategy to Improve Quality in Health Care', *European Journal of Public Health*, 15: 6–8.

Stuteley, H. and Cohen, C. (2004) 'Community Partnership for Health and Well-being: The Falmouth Beacon Project', *Journal of Integrated Care*, 12: 19–27.

WHO Centre for Health Promotion in Hospitals and Health Care. Available online at http://www.hpc-hc.cc/mission.php

World Health Organization (2007) *Schools for Health Education and Development: A Call for Action* (Geneva: WHO).

References

Addley, K., McQuillan, D. and Ruddle, M. (2001) 'Creating Healthy Workplaces in Northern Ireland: Evaluation of a Lifestyle and Physical Activity Assessment Programme', *Occupational Medicine*, 51: 439–49.

Aujoulat, I., Le Faou, A.-L., Sandrin-Berthon, B., Martin, F. and Deccache, A. (2001) 'Implementing Health Promotion in Health Care Settings: Conceptual Coherence and Policy Support', *Patient Education and Counselling*, 45: 245–54.

Aronsson, G., Gustafsson, K. and Dallner, M. (2000) 'Sick but yet at Work. An Empirical Study of Sickness Presenteeism', *Journal of Epidemiology Community Health*, 54: 502–9.

Bagnall, P. (1997) 'The Future Contribution of School Nurses to the Health of School Age Children', *Health Education*, 97: 127–31.

Bakx, J., Dietscher, C. and Visser, A. (2001) 'Editorial: "Health Promoting Hospitals"', *Patient Education and Counseling*, 45: 237–8.

Barnes, M., Courtney, M.D., Pratt, J. and Walsh, A.M. (2004) 'School-based Youth Health Nurses: Roles, Responsibilities, Challenges and Rewards', *Public Health Nursing*, 21: 316–22.

Bartley, J.D. (2004) 'Health Promotion and School Nurses: The Potential for Change', *Community Practitioner*, 77(2): 61–4.

Bensberg, M., Kennedy, M. and Bennetts, S. (2003) 'Identifying the Opportunities for Health Promoting Emergency Departments', *Accident and Emergency Nursing*, 11: 173–81.

Berg, J., Tichacek, M.J. and Theodorakis, R. (2004) 'Evaluation of an Educational Program for Adolescents with Asthma', *Journal of School Nursing*, 20: 29–35.

Carlson, G.D. and Warne, T. (2007) 'Do Healthier Nurses make Better Health Promoters? A Review of the Literature', *Nurse Education Today*, 27: 506–13.

Casey, D. (2007) 'Nurses' Perceptions, Understanding and Experiences of Health Promotion', *Journal of Clinical Nursing*, 16: 1039–49.

Chan, F.Y.S. and Wong, G.K.C. (2000) 'Health Promotion in Hospitals: The Attitudes of Health Care Professionals', *Hong Kong Nursing Journal*, 36(2): 7–15.

Chu, C., Breucker, G., Harris, N., Stitzel, A., Gan, X., Gu, X. and Dwyer, S. (2000) 'Health Promoting Workplaces – International Settings Development', *Health Promotion International*, 15: 155–67.

Cleary, M. and Walter, G. (2005) 'Towards a Healthier Lifestyle for Staff of a Psychiatric Hospital: Description of a Pilot Programme', *International Journal of Mental Health Nursing*, 14: 32–6.

Coakley, A.L. (1998) 'Health Promotion in a Hospital Ward: Reality or Asking the Impossible?', *Journal of the Royal Society of Health*, 118: 217–20.

Croghan, E., Johnson, C. and Aveyard, P. (2004) 'School Nurses: Policies, Working Practices, Roles and Value Perceptions', *Journal of Advanced Nursing*, 47: 377–85.

Cullen, A. (2002) 'Health Promotion in the Changing Face of the Hospital Landscape', *Collegian*, 9: 41–2.

Curless, M. and Burns, S. (2003) 'A Survey of Health Promotion at International Schools', *Journal of School Health*, 73(4): 133–7.

DeBell, D. and Everett, G. (1998) 'The Changing Role of School Nursing within Health Education and Health Promotion', *Health Education*, 98(3): 107–15.

DoH (1994) *Health Promoting Hospitals* (London: DoH, NHS Executive).

DoH (2004) *Choosing Health: Making Healthier Choices Easier* (London: HMSO).

Deschesnes, M., Martin, C. and Hill, A.J. (2003) 'Comprehensive Approaches to School Health Promotion: How to Achieve Broader Implementation?', *Health Promotion International*, 18: 387–96.

Dooris, M. (2001) 'The "Health Promoting University": A Critical Exploration of Theory and Practice', *Health Education*, 201(2): 51–60.

Dooris, M. (2005) 'Healthy Settings: Challenges to Generating Evidence of Effectiveness', *Health Promotion International*, 21: 55–65.

Dooris, M., Poland, B., Kolbe, L., De Leeuw, E., McCall, D.S. and Wharf-Higgins, J. (2007) 'Healthy Settings: Building Evidence for Effectiveness of Whole System Health Promotion – Challenges and Future Directions', in McQueen, D.V. and Jones, C.M. (eds), *Global Perspectives on Health Promotion Effectiveness* (New York: Springer): 327–52.

Dooris, M. and Thompson, J. (2001) 'Health-promoting Universities: An Overview', in Scriven, A. and Orme, J. (eds), *Health Promotion: Professional Perspectives* (Basingstoke: Palgrave Macmillan): 156–68.

Duke, M. and Street, M. (2003) 'Hospital in the Home: Constructions of the Nursing Role – A Literature Review', *Journal of Clinical Nursing*, 12: 852–9.

Eliason, K. and True, A. (2004) 'Combining Health Promotion Classroom Lessons with Health Fair Activities', *Journal of School Nursing*, 20: 50–3.

Ennals, R. (2002) 'Partnerships for Sustainable Healthy Workplaces', *Annals of Occupational Hygiene*, 46: 423–8.

Estabrooks, P., Dzewaltowski, D.A., Glasgow, R.E. and Klesges, L.M. (2003) 'Reporting of Validity from School Health Promotion Studies Published in 12 Leading Journals, 1996–2000', *Journal of School Health*, 73(1): 21–8.

Geiger, B.F., Mauser-Galvin, M., Cleaver, V., Petri, C.J. and Winnail, S.D. (2002) 'Working with Colleges and Universities To Enhance the Health of Students and Schools', *Health Promotion Practice*, 3: 50–9.

Germann, K. and Wilson, D. (2004) 'Organisational Capacity for Community Development in Regional Health Authorities: A Conceptual Model', *Health Promotion International*, 19: 289–98.

Goel, V. and McIsaac, W (2000) 'Health Promotion in Clinical Practice', in Poland, B.D., Green, L.W. and Rootman, I. (eds), *Settings for Health Promotion: Linking Theory and Practice* (London: Sage): 217–33.

Groene, O. (2005) 'Evaluating the Progress of the Health Promoting Hospitals Initiative?: A WHO Perspective', *Health Promotion International*, 20: 205–7.

Guilmette, T.J., Motta, S.I., Shadel, W.G., Mukand, J. and Niaura, R. (2001) 'Promoting Smoking Cessation in the Rehabilitation Setting', *American Journal of Physical and Medical Rehabilitation*, 80: 560–2.

Guo, X.H., Tian, X.Y., Pan, Y.S., Yang, X.H., Wu, S.Y., Wang, W. and Lin, V. (2007) 'Managerial Attitudes on the Development of Health Promoting Hospitals in Beijing', *Health Promotion International*, 22: 182–90.

Hampshire, M. (2003) 'To a Healthy Degree'. Available online at http://www.hda-online.org.uk/hdt/0203/universities.html (accessed 8 September 2008).

Hartrick, G., Elizabeth Lindsey, A. and Hills, M. (1994) 'Family Nursing Assessment: Meeting the Challenge of Health Promotion', *Journal of Advanced Nursing*, 20: 85–91.

Hesman, A. (2007) 'Creating Supportive Environments for Health', in Wills, J. (ed.), *Promoting Health: Vital Notes for Nurses* (Oxford: Blackwell): 175–93.

Holdsworth, M., Raymond, N.T. and Haslam, C. (2004) 'Does the Heartbeat Award Scheme in England Result in Change in Dietary Behaviour in the Workplace?', *Health Promotion International*, 19(2): 197–204.

Huyhn, K., Kosmyna, B., Lea, H., Munch, K.R., Reynolds, H.S., Specht, C., Tinker, E.C., Yee, A.J. and French, L.R. (2000) 'Creating an Adolescent Health Promotion', Internet site: 'A Community Partnership between University Nursing Students and an Inner-city High School', *Nursing and Healthcare Perspectives*, 21(3): 122–6.

Irvine, F. (2007) 'Examining the Correspondence of Theoretical and Real Interpretations of Health Promotion', *Journal of Clinical Nursing*, 16: 593–602.

Jensen, B.B. (2000) 'Health Knowledge and Health Education in the Democratic Health-promoting School', *Health Education*, 100(4): 146–54.

Joffres, C., Heath, S., Farquharson, J., Barkhouse, K., Latter, C. and MacLean, D.R. (2004) 'Facilitators and Challenges to Organisational Capacity Building in Heart Health Promotion', *Qualitative Health Research*, 14: 39–60.

Johnson, J.L. (2000) 'The Health Care Institution as a Setting for Health Promotion', in Poland, B., Green, L. and Rootman, I. (eds), *Settings for Health Promotion: Linking Theory and Practice* (London: Sage): 175–99.

Johnson, A. and Baum, F. (2001) 'Health Promotion Hospitals: A Typology of Different Organizational Approaches to Health Promotion', *Health Promotion International*, 16: 281–7.

Johnson, C.J., Croghan, E. and Crawford, J. (2003) 'The Problem and Management of Sickness Absence in the NHS: Considerations for Nurse Managers', *Journal of Nursing Management*, 11: 336–42.

Kearsey, K. (2003) 'Your Work Your Health: Whether Patient or Health Care Provider, a Healthy Workplace is Key to Well-being', *Registered Nurse Journal*, 15(1): 16–19.

Kessler, R., Ames, M., Hymel, P.A., Loeppke, R., McKenas, D.K., Richling, D.E., Stang, P.E. and Ustun, T.B. (2004) 'Using the World Health Organization Health and Work Performance Questionnaire (HPQ) to Evaluate the Indirect Workplace Costs of Illness', *Journal of Occupational and Environmental Medicine*, 46(6): S23–S37.

Konu, A. and Rimpela, M. (2002) 'Well-being in Schools: A Conceptual Mode', *Health Promotion International*, 17: 79–87.

Lalonde, M. (1989) 'Hospitals must become True Health Centres', *Dimensions*, November: 39–41.

Larsson, B. and Zaluha, M. (2003) 'Swedish School Nurses' View of School Health Care Utilisation, Causes and Management of Recurrent Headaches among School Children', *Scandanavian Journal of Caring Sciences*, 17: 232–8.

Lee, A., Tsang, K.-K., Lee, S.-H., To, C.-Y. and Kwan, T.-F. (2001) 'Challenges in the Development of Health-promoting Schools: A Review of Hong Kong Innovations and Initiatives', *Health Education*, 101(2): 83–9.

Levy, S.R., Baldyga, W. and Jurkowski, J.M. (2003) 'Developing Community Health Promotion Interventions: Selecting Partners and Fostering Collaboration', *Health Promotion Practice*, 4: 314–22.

Mäenpää, T., Paavilainen. E. and Åstedt-Kurki, P. (2007) 'Cooperation with School Nurses described by Finnish Sixth-graders', *International Journal of Nursing Practice*, 13: 304–9.

Maughan, E. (2003) 'The Impact of School Nursing on School Performance: A Research Synthesis', *Journal of School Nursing*, 19: 163–71.

Maurana, C.A., Beck, B., Newton, G.L. (1998) 'How Principles of Partnership are applied to the Development of a Community–Campus Partnership', *Partnership Perspectives*, 1: 47–53.

Mavor, T. (2001) 'Like Parent, Like Child: A Health Promoting Hospital Project', *Patient Education and Counselling*, 45: 261–4.

McGhan, S.L., Reutter, L.I., Hessel, P.A., Melvin, D. and Wilson D.R. (2002) 'Developing a School Asthma Policy', *Public Health Nursing*, 19: 112–23.

Palmer, A. (2003) 'Whistle-stop Tour of the Theory and Practice of Stress Management and Preventions: Its Possible Role in Postgraduate Health Promotion', *Health Education Journal*, 62: 133–42.

Pelikan, J.M., Krajic, K. and Dietscher, C. (2001) 'The Health Promoting Hospital (HPH): Concept and Development', *Patient Education and Counselling*, 45: 239–43.

Peterson, J., Atwood, J.R. and Yates, B. (2002) 'Key Elements for Church-based Health Promotion Programs: Outcome-based Literature Review', *Public Health Nursing*, 19: 401–11.

Pelikan, J., Lobnig, H. and Krajic, K. (1997) 'Health-promoting Hospitals', *World Health*, 3: 24–5.

Petkeviciene, J., Miseviciene, I., and Petrauskas, D. (2002) 'Health Behaviour and Interest in Health Promotion in Relation to Subject of Study among Students of Kaunas Universities', *European Journal of Public Health*, 12 (supplement): 27.

Plews, C., Billingham, K. and Rowe, A. (2000) 'Public Health Nursing: Barriers and Opportunities', *Health and Social Care in the Community*, 8: 138–46.

Poland, B., Green, L. and Rootman, I. (2000) *Settings for Health Promotion: Linking Theory and Practice* (London: Sage).

Põlluste, K., Alop, J., Groene, O., Härm, T., Merisalu, E. and Suurorg, L. (2007) 'Health-promoting Hospitals in Estonia: What Are They Doing Differently?, *Health Promotion International*, 22: 327–36.

Quinn, J., Sengupta, S. and Cleary, H. (2001) 'The Challenge of Effectively Addressing Tobacco Control within a Health Promoting NHS Trust', *Patient Education and Counselling*, 45: 255–9.

Reger, B., Williams, K., Kolar, M., Smith, H. and Douglas, W.J. (2002) 'Implementing University-based Wellness: A Participatory Planning Approach', *Health Promotion Practice*, 3: 507–14.

Runciman, P., Watson, H., McIntosh, J. and Tolson, D. (2006) 'Community Nurses' Health Promotion Work with Older People', *Journal of Advanced Nursing*, 55: 46–57.

Rustler, C. (2002) 'Health Promoting in Hospitals. The German Network of Health Promotion in Hospitals Needs a New Accent', *Pflege Aktuell*, 56: 202–5.

Schofield, M.J., Lynagh, M. and Mishra, G. (2003) 'Evaluation of a Health Promoting Schools program to Reduce Smoking in Australian Secondary Schools', *Health Education Research*, 18: 678–92.

Scriven, A. and Stiddard, L. (2003) 'Empowering Schools: Translating Health Promotion Principles into Practice', *Health Education*, 103(2): 110–18.

Shain, M. and Kramer, D.M. (2004) 'Health Promotion in the Workplace: Framing the Concept; Reviewing the Evidence', *Occupational and Environmental Medicine*, 61: 643–8.

Smith, A.B., Gaffney, M. and Nairn, K. (2004) 'Health Rights in Secondary Schools: Student and Staff Perspectives', *Health Education Research*, 19: 85–97.

Starfield, B. (2001) 'New Paradigms for Quality in Primary Care', *British Journal of General Practice*, 51: 303–9.

Stears, D. (1998) 'Evaluating *The Implementation of the European Network of Health Promoting Schools* in Six European Countries', *Health Education*, 98(5): 173–81.

Stock, C., Wille, L. and Kramer, A. (2001) 'Gender-specific Health Behaviours of German University Students Predict the Interest in Campus Health Promotion', *Health Promotion International*, 16: 145–54.

Sun, J. and Stewart, D. (2007) 'How Effective is the Health-promoting Schools Approach in Building Social Capital in Primary Schools?', *Health Education*, 107: 556–74.

Thome, B., Dykes, A.-K. and Hallberg, L.R. (2003) 'Home Care with Regard to Definition, Care Recipients, Content and Outcome: Systematic Literature Review', *Journal of Clinical Nursing*, 12: 860–72.

Thomson, P. and Kohli, H. (1997) 'Health Promotion Training Needs Analysis: An Integrated Role for Clinical Nurses in Lanarkshire, Scotland', *Journal of Advanced Nursing*, 26: 507–14.

Tossavainen, K., Turunen, H., Jakonen, S., Tupala, M. and Vertio, H. (2004) 'School Nurses as Health Counsellors in Finnish ENHPS Schools', *Health Education*, 104(1): 33–44.

Tsouros, A., Dowding, G., Thompson, J. and Dooris, M. (1998) *Health Promoting Universities: Concept, Experience and Framework for Action* (Copenhagen: WHO Regional Office for Europe).

Turunen, H., Tossavainen, K., Jakonen, S., Salomaki, U. and Vertio, H. (2002) 'Improving Health in the European Network of Health Promoting Schools in Finland', *Health Education*, 100(6): 252–60.

Verow, P. and Hargreaves, C. (2000) 'Healthy Workplace Indicators: Costing Reasons for Sickness Absence within the UK National Health Service', *Occupational Medicine*, 50(4): 251–7.

Wainwright, P., Thomas, J. and Jones, M. (2000) 'Health Promotion and the Role of the School Nurse: A Systematic Review', *Journal of Advanced Nursing*, 32: 1083–91.

Wass, A. (2000) *Promoting Health: The Primary Health Care Approach*, 2nd edn (Sydney, Australia: Harcourt).

Watson, M. (2008) 'Going for Gold: The Health Promoting General Practice', *Quality in Primary Care*, 16: 177–85.

Watson, R., Stimpson, A., and Hostick, T. (2004) 'Prison Health Care: A Review of the Literature', *International Journal of Nursing Studies*, 41: 119–224.

Weare, K. (2002) 'The Contribution of Education to Health Promotion', in Bunton, R. and Macdonald, G. (eds), *Health Promotion: Disciplines, Diversity and Developments*, 2nd edn (London: Routledge): 102–25.

Weil, P. and Harmata, R. (2002) 'Rekindling the Flame: Routine Practices that Promote Hospital Community Leadership', *Journal of Health Care Management*, 47(2): 98–109.

Whitehead, D. (2004a) 'Health Promoting Universities (HPU): The Role and Function of Nursing', *Nurse Education Today*, 24: 466–72.

Whitehead, D. (2004b) 'The European Health Promoting Hospitals (HPH) Project – How Far On?', *Health Promotion International*, 19: 259–67.

Whitehead, D. (2005) Health Promoting Hospitals (HPH): The Role and Function of Nursing', *Journal of Clinical Nursing*, 14: 20–7.

Whitehead, D. (2006a) 'Health Promoting Prisons (HPP) and the Imperative for Nursing', *International Journal of Nursing Studies*, 43: 123–31.

Whitehead, D. (2006b) The Health Promoting School (HPS): What Role for Nursing?', *Journal of Clinical Nursing*, 15: 264–71.

Whitehead, D. (2006c) 'Workplace Health Promotion: The Role and Responsibilities of Nursing Managers', *Journal of Nursing Management*, 14: 59–68.

Whitehead, D. and Russell, G. (2004) 'How Effective are Health Education Programmes: Resistance, Reactance, Rationality and Risk? Recommendations for Effective Practice', *International Journal of Nursing Studies*, 41: 163–72.

WHO (1986) *Ottawa Charter for Health Promotion* (Ottawa: WHO).

WHO (1991) *The Budapest Declaration of Health Promoting Hospitals* (Copenhagen: WHO).

WHO (1995a) *Global Strategy on Occupational Health for All: The Way to Health at Work. Recommendation of the Second Meeting of the WHO Collaborating Centres in Occupational Health – 1994, Beijing, China* (Geneva: WHO).

WHO (1995b) *WHO Expert Committee on Comprehensive School Health Education and Health Promotion* (Geneva: WHO).

WHO (1997) *The Vienna Recommendations on Health Promoting Hospitals* (Copenhagen: WHO).

WHO (2003) 'Health Promoting Hospitals'. Available online at http://www.euro.who.int/healthpromo-hosp (accessed 25 September 2008).

WHO (2008) 'Promoting Health and Safety at the Workplace'. Available at www.euro.who.int/Document/EEHC/26th_EEHC_Madrid_edoc08rev1.pdf – 2008-10-17 (accessed 9 September 2008).

Wilkinson, E., Elander, E. and Woolaway, M. (1997) 'Exploring the Use of Action Research to Stimulate and Evaluate Workplace Health Promotion', *Health Education Journal*, 56: 188–98.

Wright, J., Franks, A., Ayres, P., Jones, K., Roberts, T. and Whitty, P. (2002) 'Public Health in Hospitals: The Missing Link in Health Improvement', *Journal of Public Health Medicine*, 24(3): 152–5.

Xiangyang, T., Lan, Z., Xueping, M., Tao, Z, Yuzhen, S. and Jagusztyn, M. (2003) 'Beijing Health Promoting Universities: Practice and Evaluation', *Health Promotion International*, 18: 107–13.

CHAPTER 6

Evidence Based Practice in Health Promotion

Sean Mackay

Objectives:

By the end of this chapter you should be able to:

- Define evidence based practice in the context of health promotion
- Discuss the link between evidence based practice and research
- Consider a range of research methodologies and their usefulness for health promotion
- Identify barriers to evidence based health promotion and their possible solutions

---

Key terms

- Evidence based practice (EBP)
- Health promotion evidence
- Qualitative research
- Quantitative research
- Research methodology
- Research process

Introduction

Evidence based practice (EBP) informs a number of key decision-makers in health promotion, including practitioners, managers, purchasers; and the clients and community that are subject to health promotion interventions (South and Tilford 2000; Gerrish et al. 2007). In today's health care climate, there is an expectation that health interventions are justified by demonstrating the tangible benefits of different approaches. For example, the UK's Department of Health (DoH) clearly states that targets set by primary care trusts should be evidence based (DoH 2004: 86, 91) and that, in particular, preventative services for older people should be evidence based, (DoH 2006: 30), as should local mental health promotion interventions (DoH 2006: 39). Ensuring health promotion is evidence based, through such legislation, should then facilitate the effective use of resources – although other factors might impede this, such as financial constraints or the decision-makers' own experience (Elliot and Popay 2000). Similarly, when resources are scarce, as is often the case with most health services, interventions that are not supported by evidence might become low priority (Rada et al. 1999).

This chapter will discuss definitions of evidence based practice, and give examples of a range of research methodologies that can be used to develop the evidence base of health promotion. The complex nature of some health promotion interventions, or the complexity of the setting in which they are being applied, raises issues that impact on the application of evidence based health promotion. These issues will be explored and a model is presented to illustrate how evidence bases relate to the health promotion processes discussed in earlier chapters. Finally, barriers to implementing evidence based health promotion are discussed and possible solutions put forward.

What is evidence based practice (EBP) and evidence based health promotion (EBHP)?

The World Health Organization (WHO) clearly set out definitions of health promotion in the *Ottawa Charter* (WHO 1986) and the *Jakarta Declaration* (WHO 1997). Furthermore, the WHO produced a glossary of terms relating to health promotion in 1986 – further revising it in 1998 (WHO 1998b). However, they were slow to characterize EBHP, and took until 2006 to produce the following definition of EBHP. For them, EBHP is:

> The use of information derived from formal research and systematic investigation to identify causes and contributing factors to health needs and the most effective health promotion actions to address these in given contexts and populations. (Smith et al. 2006)

In light of this definition, it can be surmised that evidence might be based on research or other systematic investigation to enable health promotion practitioners, including nurses, to assess what works, what evidence demonstrates that it works, and the strength of the evidence.

The concept of EBHP has developed from the understanding of evidence based medicine (EBM). The classic definition of this was offered by Sackett et al. (1996: 72) as:

> Evidence based medicine is the conscientious, explicit, and judicious use of current best evidence in making decisions about the care of individual patients.

In other words, creating an evidence base for practice involves the painstaking, clear, wise and open use of *proof* or *truth* to inform care provision. The issue of what constitutes truth or proof will be examined later in this chapter. Rada et al. (1999) paraphrase Sackett et al.'s (1996) definition to embrace health promotion, and add that health promotion interventions can be aimed at communities and populations. Thus, they contend that EBHP is about integrating local expertise with 'the best available external evidence yielded by systematic research' (Rada et al. 1999: 178). Sackett and his colleagues later went on to revise their definition of EBM to include not only best evidence and local professional expertise, but also patients' values and opinions too. South and Tilford (2000) identify that health promotion specialists draw on their own knowledge and expertise as to what is accepted as 'good practice' and appropriate health promotion theory, to add to the evidence they present for their own practice. This suggests that internal evidence has a part to play in EBHP. Authors such as Cornwall (1996) also refer to local evidence: what counts as local evidence is explored later in this chapter.

Evidence based practice is generally accepted as a 'good thing' (Perkins et al. 1999). Evidence facilitates effective use of resources and strategy development (Rada 1999), identifies the 'best way' to promote health (WHO 2007), and demonstrates the worth of health promotion activity for policy-makers and for the wider community (Rychetnik and Wise 2004). However, Seedhouse (1996) reminds us that values also drive health promotion practice. Indeed, the use of theoretical models to underpin practice can allow analysis of the underlying values that relate to certain health promotion approaches. Seedhouse (1996) does warn that, if health promoters focus on evidence in preference to values, it removes the political element of health promotion – such as empowerment, participation and poverty-reduction – and runs the risk of over-simplifying health promotion In this scenario, the wider determinants of health might not be considered and health, as the absence of disease rather than the concept of *well-being*, could become the goal of health promotion.

Research and evidence based practice

The link between EBHP and research needs to be considered. Bowling (2002: 1) defines research as:

> the systematic and rigorous process of enquiry which aims to describe phenomena and to develop and test explanatory concepts and theories.

However, McVicar (1999: 299) distinguishes between two aspects of research: *doing research* – discovering, developing and testing knowledge; and *reading* or *critiquing research* – accessing scientific knowledge for practice. For nurses who want to deliver EBHP, it would appear appropriate for both activities to be undertaken.

Health promotion evaluation is defined elsewhere in this book (see Chapter 4). Much is written on the subject, but Feuerstein (1986: 2), in the opening of her seminal book on evaluating health-promoting community development programmes, defines the process of evaluation as 'to assess the value of something'. If a health promotion intervention has been evaluated as worthwhile, then this could be considered valuable for others wishing to find appropriate methods of working. In this context, evaluation should be considered a useful source of evidence for EBHP. However, a report for the UK's Kings Fund by Coote et al. (2004: xi), on reviewing what actually works in community-based initiatives – such as Sure Start – conclude that:

> Complex, community-based initiatives are hard to evaluate because of their size and the speed with which they are being rolled out, and because they are trying to address multiple problems within shifting political environments.

Similarly, O'Dwyer et al.'s (2007) systematic review of area based initiatives, using a variety of strategies aimed at areas rather than individuals or social groups to tackle health inequalities, reported that many studies were unable to demonstrate cause and effect when evaluating the effectiveness of interventions – in part, because the strategies were used in combination. Therefore, it might prove difficult for complex community health promotion interventions to generate straightforward evidence that is unequivocal, despite the need for such evidence. Nurses and other health practitioners seeking the evidence base for this type of intervention will need to bear this in mind when appraising evidence.

It is important to unpick the terms 'research' and 'evaluation' in relation to evidence and evidence based practice. Perhaps this is best illustrated by the debate on research versus practice. In particular, it is noteworthy that the standards that define good research are different to those that define good practice (Learmonth 2000). Tilford (2000) explains that the main aim of researchers is to contribute to the evidence base for a discipline, without necessarily being concerned with the needs of the users of that evidence (that is, the practitioner). Although health promotion practitioners might carry out research for the purposes of evaluation (Learmonth 2000; South and Tilford 2000), the aim of evaluation is not necessarily to generate new evidence; rather, it is to identify what has come out of a specific project. South and Tilford (2000: 732) identify some key perceived differences between research and evaluation based on their own interviews with health promotion specialists. They suggest that practitioners perceive research to be a larger scale exercise with broad research questions examined in a more focused, structured and academically rigorous way. On the other hand, evaluation was considered smaller scale, less structured and less focused, with narrower questions that are looked at in less depth. Evaluation is seen as an everyday activity for health promotion specialists, unlike the occasional research project. It is also perceived that research, in this context, would more likely be generalizable, would produce academic papers and would need help from beyond the individual health promoter to be achieved. If the view is taken that evaluation is not considered sufficiently extensive or methodo-logically rigorous to contribute to the evidence base, this precludes the use of 'real world' evidence (Nutbeam 1996) – which is generated by health promoters evaluating their own practice, and which might still be more valuable to inform their peers than academic research. With this stance, health promoters, as nurses, run the risk of disregarding much evidence that could be of value in informing their own practice.

Other forms of evidence

Rycroft-Malone et al. (2004) identify a number of other useful sources of evidence including:

- That which is based on professional practice and might be intuitive: they argue that, ideally, such evidence should be disseminated and critiqued for verification
- A sense of individual or collective meaning based on experience
- Evidence derived from the local context in which the intervention is carried out

Therefore, evidence from these sources is dynamic, eclectic and depends on the context, and so, as such, is not fixed or certain. Those who seek a single or 'fixed' truth are likely to be disappointed. At the same time, it is worth noting that this is the nature of health promotion – operating in inherently complex environments (Jackson and Waters 2005) (see Chapter 1). If this is the case, nurses need to maintain a 'wide screen view' of what constitutes evidence and draw on a wide range of types of evidence to inform their practice. This is covered in the next section of this chapter.

What counts as evidence?

Health promotion, as discussed throughout this book, is an activity that uses multiple interventions to achieve outcomes related to complex phenomena – such as improvements in social capital, community empowerment and reductions in health inequalities. Therefore, measuring whether or not health promotion has been successful in itself is likely to be problematic or, at the very least, complex. Yet, nurses wanting to plan effective health promotion practice, or to demonstrate that their activity has been effective, are required to be able to use the evidence base of health promotion. Once strongly held ideologies and values are taken into account, along with cross-sectoral partnerships and the involvement of the community in health promotion interventions, it is not surprising that what counts as evidence remains highly contested (Wimbush and Watson 2000).

Generally speaking, research can be categorized into two main paradigms (theoretical worldviews): *quantitative* and *qualitative*. Quantitative research aims to ensure that the findings are unbiased (objective), reliable and generalizable to a wider population – collecting numerical information (data) and using a range of statistical tests to analyze the data (Bowling 2002). In contrast, qualitative research seeks the meaning attached to people's experiences, beliefs, feelings or perceptions – where reality might be interpreted differently and subjectively (Polit and Beck 2006; Macnee and McCabe 2008). Qualitative data is collected in the form of words, not numbers, which cannot be statistically manipulated or generalized to a wider population.

In the Western scientific paradigm, there is considered to be a hierarchy of evidence (Evans 2003; and see Figure 6.1), which is supported by the *BMJ* and the *Cochrane Library* – as well as a range of clinical guideline groups throughout the world. In the hierarchy, some types of evidence are considered to be more valuable than other evidence and these decisions are based on levels of likely bias, risk of

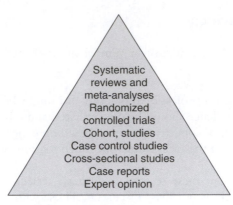

Figure 6.1 Hierarchy of research evidence

error, validity and generalizability associated with different methodological approaches. The research design – classically and traditionally considered as the 'gold standard' (that is, the best, most robust and reliable for a single study) – is the randomized controlled trial (RCT). Evans (2003) warns that a hierarchy should only be considered a guide to judge the strength of evidence, measured by its effectiveness (did the intervention work?). It is clear that issues such as feasibility and appropriateness need also to be considered. It should be noted that the hierarchy of evidence presented below generally refers to quantitative approaches (with the exception of 'expert opinion'). The relevance of hierarchies to qualitative approaches will be discussed in a later section of this chapter.

Additional point

Validity and reliability are two key terms that are used in quantitative research. Validity is the level of accuracy of the measure being used, and reliability is the level of consistency. For example, in a set of questions in a questionnaire to measure risk of post natal depression, the reliability indicates whether answers would change depending on the person administering the questionnaire, and validity would indicate how accurately the tool would predict the risk of post natal depression. Generalizability is the likelihood that findings from a piece of research can be applied to a wider population than the population being tested.

Systematic review and meta-analyses are approaches that take an overview of evidence from a variety of experimental designs, the most favoured being the RCT. Therefore, first, it is useful to establish what an RCT is, and then look at systematic reviews and meta-analyses in a little more depth. The other types of evidence are summarized in Table 6.1.

Table 6.1 Other methodologies indicated within the research hierarchy of evidence

Methodology	Brief description	Strengths	Limitations	Relevance to HP
Cohort studies	A trend study that focuses on a particular sub-population from which data are collected at different points over a period of time.	Allows data to be collected at intervals and captures any changes that take place over time	High risk of attrition where individual participants drop out of the study for various reasons, thus compromising the generalizability of findings	Useful to capture how attitudes beliefs and behaviours change over time (for example, changes in attitudes to drink driving)
Case control studies	A descriptive method that compares the characteristics of the subject group (who have been exposed to a risk factor, or those with a specific condition) with a control or reference group	Seeks to investigate cause and effect: do some factors occur more frequently in the case group?	Need to recruit from population of interest for both case and control groups – might lead to problems in sampling. Retrospective approach might lead to recall bias from participants.	Mainly used for identifying possible risk factors leading to certain conditions Could be useful in field of accident prevention
Cross-sectional studies	A descriptive study of a representative sample (cross-section) of the population of interest at a point in time	Might be used to identify people of interest, who are then investigated in further detail	Is only a snapshot at that particular time, therefore might be of limited generalizability in the future	Useful to explore the link between variables in a population (e.g. time watching TV and taking exercise in adolescent males – Chen et al. 2008)
Case report	Presentation of findings from a single client	Might raise some issues or questions for further research or study	Very low generalizability, as findings based on one subject	Questionable relevance for individual, but might be useful if case is a community or population, (e.g. report on intervention to change community perception of diabetes) (Bisset et al. 2004)
Expert opinion	Views of respected authority on the subject, based on experience from practice, reports of findings of expert committees	Not necessarily bound by the usual constraints (e.g. ethics, cost) of experimental research	Who is an expert?	Might be useful to capture a new standpoint, take stock of the current situation, or suggest a direction of travel for health promoters

The randomized controlled trial (RCT)

This experimental design has been developed from natural science, and has achieved high status within the hierarchy of evidence because it fits predominantly within a positivist biomedical model of health (see Chapter 2). Positivism uses quantitative methods to generate evidence that is based on observation and measurement. RCT's are useful when it is possible to assign individuals randomly between an experimental group (or groups), whose members receive the intervention being tested, and a control group, whose members usually receive a placebo. The outcomes of the two groups are compared. This process might be blind, where the participants and even the investigators (double-blind) do not know to which group individuals have been assigned (Bowling 2002). The role of the participant in this type of research is as a passive responder to the experimental intervention.

The purpose of the RCT is, therefore, to study cause and affect relationships between variables. In health promotion, the RCT might have some uses in researching or evaluating the effectiveness of interventions such as individual behavioural change initiatives; for example, in tackling smoking in school children.

Health promotion in action

A randomized controlled trial (Stephenson et al. 2004), investigating pupil led (peer) sex education in schools, randomized schools into an intervention group – where pupil peer educators were trained, in addition to the schools' usual sex and relationships education (SRE), and a control group – where only the schools' usual SRE input was delivered. As well as reported levels of unprotected first intercourse before the age of 16 years, the researchers also measured other factors – such as quality of relationship with partner, satisfaction with sex education and knowledge levels about STI (sexually transmitted infection) prevention, confidence and behaviour, measured by questionnaire. Observation and focus groups were also carried out. Follow-up was completed at 6-month and 18-month intervals after the intervention, and the incidence of termination of pregnancy by 19–20 years was measured. Analysis demonstrated greater satisfaction with SRE in the pupil led groups, and modest differences in unprotected first sexual intercourse for girls. The authors raise questions about the most appropriate method of selecting peer educators, and note that single-sex groups for the sessions would have been preferred by the pupils.

However, it is often argued that experimental research is in contradiction to key values of health promotion, such as empowerment and participation, where personal experience is an important element. RCTs are not interested in exploring personal perspectives. Indeed, the WHO (1998a) suggests that RCTs are inappropriate and misleading when used to measure the effectiveness of health promotion interventions, not to mention how expensive they usually are to conduct. The research undertaken by Stephenson et al. (2004), however, moves beyond this, as it used qualitative methods as well as the ascertaining of pupils' views on their satisfaction with peer led sex and relationship education. Thus, they also consider the important subjective elements of the intervention. RCTs work best for single-factor interventions, or where there is a direct relationship between intervention and outcome (Nutbeam 2000), and so often are not the best method for complex health promotion interventions. Furthermore, within a health promotion context there is a risk of 'leakage' between the control and experimental group, and the difficulty around gaining informed consent raises further ethical issues (Nutbeam et al. 1993; Learmonth and Watson 1999).

Systematic reviews

The systematic review is a research design that is highly valued as a resource for evidence based practice and, as such, sits at the top of the hierarchy of evidence. A systematic review addresses a specific question from practice by methodically drawing together high quality research literature on that subject and summarizing the findings of these studies (Mcnee and McCabe 2008). Systematic reviews do not statistically analyze the data from the individual studies, but they do have strict inclusion criteria. Because multiple studies are considered, systematic reviews are less likely to provide misleading findings than an individual study.

Health promotion in action

Thomas and Perera (2006) carried out a systematic review of school based smoking cessation programmes and, in particular, whether classroom sessions could reduce the uptake of smoking in the long term. The authors searched for and reviewed randomized controlled trials for school based behavioural interventions for children and adolescents. However, one of the inclusion criteria was that individuals, classes, schools or districts were randomized into intervention or control groups (that is, the control group would not receive the programme). The study identified 94 RCTs, but only 23 were identified as sufficiently robust to be included in the systematic review. The review revealed that there was no strong evidence of the long-term effects of the intervention, but that there was limited evidence of success where 'developing generic social competence' was included, or when the intervention included community approaches.

Systematic reviews are a useful source for practitioners wishing to implement EBHP. However, while systematic reviews are useful in presenting a summary of research findings on a particular health promotion topic, systematic reviews rely on the hierarchy of evidence, favouring positivist quantitative methodologies over all others (Learmonth 2000; Stewart-Brown 2001). For instance, in the offered example of Thomas and Perera (2006), only studies with randomization of controls were included. For health promoters wishing to implement a smoking prevention programme in a school, it might prove impractical for pupils to receive the interventions in isolation from those who receive no intervention (the controls) over the study period. With any group or population, there is always the danger of 'contamination' amongst the respondents whereby the controls could indirectly receive the intervention without this being known.

Focusing on quantitative studies for systematic reviews might lead to under-reporting of findings of health promotion initiatives that are researched using methods perhaps more appropriate to the subject matter (for example, qualitative methodologies). Similarly, there might be a disproportionate focus on simpler inter-ventions that might lend themselves to be more readily researched using quantita-tive approaches, meaning that they are less relevant to practising health promotion in the real world. Howes et al. (2004) identify possible 'publication bias' with systematic reviews relating to EBHP. They point out that much of the health promo-tion research does not appear in the public domain and is hard to locate. For example, findings might not be published in peer reviewed journals but, instead, appear in doctoral theses and organizational reports and so on (the so called 'grey literature'). Selection and inclusion criteria for systematic reviews might exclude non-English language journals, or those with lower methodological quality. Research that demonstrates a significantly negative result is less likely to be published than research demonstrating significantly positive results (Torgerson 2006). These publi-cation biases might affect the results of systematic reviews and meta-analyses. In the attempt to be as accurate as possible, the full picture might not be presented.

Other methodologies

Table 6.1 lists the other methodologies, other than the previously discussed RCTs and systematic reviews indicated within the hierarchy of evidence, and gives an over-view of their strengths and possible limitations, as well as their possible relevance to health promotion.

Qualitative approaches

An alternative to quantitative positivist approaches for nurses to use is a range of qualitative approaches to produce evidence for nurses' health promotion practice. Currently, it is fair to say that the majority of nursing based research comes under the umbrella of the qualitative paradigm. Qualitative methodologies take a relativist – rather than positivist – approach, searching for relative meaning in their findings, as meanings, perceptions and experiences are sought from participants.

McQueen (2001) argues that there is no consensus on the hierarchy of evidence for community research. This might be compounded when nurses pursue a health promotion aim, working in the community and being guided by that community, since they follow an unpredictable course (Baum 1995). However, Daly et al. (2007) assert that policy-makers need a way to judge the quality and value of qualitative studies to weigh up the evidence base, suggesting that decision-makers value evidence or findings that are transferable to other settings. Instead of attaching names to qualitative research methods, as in the hierarchy of quantitative methods, Daly et al. (2007) identify four types of study. These range from *single-case studies, descriptive studies* (of groups of participants) and *conceptual studies* (where sample selection was influenced by a conceptual or theoretical framework) through to, at the top of the hierarchy, *generalizable studies*, which include a full account of the data collection and analysis, and where issues of generalizability are explored in a review of the literature. They point out that the limitation of this type of report, for publication, is its size. If all the detail were put into the report, it would be too large to publish.

Health promotion in action

Jamieson et al. (2007) used focus groups to ascertain the understanding, attitudes and beliefs about oral health in a disadvantaged group. In this case, it was indigenous Australians who, as a collective population, generally experience poor oral health. The researchers believed that other more rigid data collection methods would be less likely to reveal cultural factors influencing self-care behaviours. They recruited a range of participants from local health and non-health groups, and identified several themes – including post-colonial dietary changes and the difference in principles of the Western model of health services and the indigenous cultural principle of holism. They used their findings to develop culturally appropriate oral health initiatives.

So, while there is not the commonly accepted hierarchy of evidence in qualitative research in the way that there is in quantitative research, there are elements of study design or reporting in publication that affect the value of qualitative evidence. Perhaps a little worryingly, Wilhelmsson and Lindberg (2007) note in their literature review of EBHP in primary care that few studies into prevention and health promotion in primary care were of a high scientific quality, especially where the focus was on the role of the nurse. These studies tended to be of a descriptive design. The authors noted:

> Presumably, nurses do a great deal of preventive work, but it is not documented and published. Nurses do not have a long tradition of systematizing and disseminating the results of their work, which is probably one explanation. (Wilhelmsson and Lindberg 2007: 264)

Nurses should not be discouraged by such findings, though. Nursing is a neophyte profession still when it comes to health promotion practice, so it is still at liberty to mould and shape its own evidence base while, at the same time, being able to draw on existing hierarchies of general health promotion evidence. Nurses should work towards disseminating evidence from their own health promotion activities in order to develop the evidence base on nurse led health promotion. Barriers and possible solutions to this approach are discussed later in this chapter. Additionally, a process of 'triangulation' could be adopted, where findings from one source of evidence are matched against other sources or methods (Denzin 1989). This activity comes under the umbrella of 'mixed methods' research, where mixing and marrying different types of methodologies, designs and data assist in providing a 'fuller picture' of events (Whitehead and Elliott 2007). When findings are confirmed by a mix of methods and sources, the level of uncertainty about a particular finding is reduced.

Participatory research

One key aspect of qualitative research, as it is used to explore the meaning and experience of people, is the role of the person or group in research. Ideally, these participants are not simply filling in questionnaires, but are actively involved in defining the research question and the methods by to answer it. This leads us to consider participatory research (usually 'action research') and its value in EBHP. The National Institute for Clinical Excellence (NICE 2008: 43) offers the following definition of participatory research:

> Participatory research is a collaborative process whereby people are encouraged to define the problems and issues of concern. They are also encouraged to help gather and analyze data and apply the research findings.

Action research, described as a *style* rather than a specific *method* of research (Meyer 2000) is participatory, democratic and seeks social change alongside the addition of scientific knowledge. Therefore, the research process can have its own positive benefits for the groups or communities undertaking it. Participatory rural appraisal (PRA), originally used in developing countries and based on the work of Paulo Freire (1972), would be considered a type of action research. This method can be useful to allow two-way learning and incorporate (and validate) local or indigenous knowledge (Cornwall 1996). That said, Cornwall warns that the level of participation of local people might range from cooption (where people are chosen to be involved but have no real input) and compliance (outsiders allocate tasks to the local people) to co-learning (local people and outsiders share knowledge, creating new understanding) and collective action (the agenda is set by the local people and they act together to carry it out). A range of techniques might be used within this paradigm, including drawing, maps and drama, and improving self-confidence in the participants who might be traditionally marginalized and without a voice. There is a danger of these processes raising expectations of local community members to a level that the researchers might not be able to fulfil. However, involving lay people in the research process (in either planning, data collecting or data analysis) might develop local skills, raise local capacity, and even empower the community to carry out further research in the future (El Ansari 2005).

Health promotion in action

Ravelsloot et al. (2007) investigated the impact of health promotion interventions on independent living for people with a disability. The authors carried out a programme of participatory action research (PAR). A group of people with disabilities and people who provide services for them developed a 'surveillance instrument' to identify prevalence and severity of limitation due to a range of conditions. The researchers originally planned to conduct individually focused health education in peoples homes as their intervention, however, the participants identified that this would exacerbate the isolation often felt by people with disabilities, opting instead for group-based interventions. The groups then developed a programme covering topics such as goal setting and nutrition. The surveillance instrument was then used to measure the effectiveness of the programme. Therefore, the participants were involved in defining the context and content of the health promotion programme, and in the measurement of its effectiveness, which generated quantitative data suitable for statistical analysis.

The debate about professional knowledge versus lay knowledge

There is a tension between the experimental, medical science driven evidence – which is valued highly in the positivist paradigm of the health service, and the health promotion ideology of community/consumer driven approaches, which values the importance of local knowledge and experience (Springett et al. 2007; Popay and Williams 1996). This tension, between professional knowledge and lay knowledge, and their methodological approaches, needs to be overcome in order to provide a greater understanding of current public health problems. For example, lay perspectives on risk will influence people's justification of smoking, developing resilience to health promotion interventions (Katainen 2006). With particular reference to smoking cessation services, Springett et al. (2007) argue that, rather than outside professionals with different experience and cultural norms, the best people to provide cessation support are those from similar circumstances as the disadvantaged groups who are considered 'hard to reach'.

Health promotion in action

Springett et al. (2007) carried out a process evaluation of the smoking cessation service in Liverpool, UK, using a combination of interviews, observations and focus groups in order to identify characteristics of the programme that contributed to its success. They identified the flexibility and accessibility of the service (so that it was client led for referral and attendance) and the fact that support was provided by lay advisors (rather than professionals) was important. The approach had been based on the personal, local experience of the lay health advisors, rather than on evidence from RCTs. However, as it became established, the project came under pressure to evaluate its work using quantitative measures to demonstrate how it effectively achieves the required outcomes for continued funding. However, evaluation methodology should be dictated by the intervention (Nutbeam 2000).

 Tutorial brief 6.1

Identify the strengths and limitations of involving lay advisors in defining the approach of a smoking cessation service.

Health promotion in action

Rhodes et al. (2007) compiled a qualitative review of the benefits in using lay health advisors for a range of health promotion interventions among Hispanics and Latinos in the USA. They reviewed 37 studies and drew out six main roles for them:

1. Supporting participant recruitment and data collection,
2. Serving as health advisors and referral sources,
3. Distributing materials,
4. Being role models,
5. Advocating on behalf of community members, and
6. Serving as co-researchers in participatory research models

Rhodes et al. (2007: 425)

This set of possible roles demonstrates that there is a range of activities with differing levels of participation for lay people in health promotion interventions. As the level of involvement increases from basic tasks to decision-making, so does their level of empowerment.

What to measure: process or outcome?

Much of the evidence published relating to health promotion considers the outcome of interventions. These might be short-term – for example, reported increase in physical exercise or reducing alcohol consumption, or long-term – such as reduction in teenage pregnancy rates or sustained smoking-cessation. Focusing on single outcome measures might lead to an over emphasis on individual behaviour-change and so is not appropriate for interventions seeking broader changes – such as interventions taking a healthy settings approach (see Chapter 5). Speller et al. (1997) argue that studies included in systematic reviews are selected on the quality of research, not the quality of the health promotion intervention. Therefore, health promotion interventions that are effective but do not meet the high standards of inclusion for research publication will not be disseminated widely. Similarly, because reports on successful interventions are more likely to be submitted and published than reports on unsuccessful health promotion interventions, lessons will not be learned from interventions that perhaps failed to achieve the planned outcome. Both of these limitations will dilute the richness of the evidence base for health promotion. So, instead of evaluating a health promotion programme by measuring whether the *outcomes* were met, *process* evaluation is a useful approach; also, any successes can be replicated (Nutbeam 2000). This type of evaluation (often using qualitative approaches) considers questions such as 'Was the process carried out as intended?', 'Were there other factors that affected the result?' (for example, the conditions that help health-promoting schools to flourish) (Inchley et al. 2006), and 'What were the participants' views of the intervention?' Parry Langdon et al. (2003: 215) argue that:

An outcome evaluation merely establishes that an intervention has worked: it contributes nothing on the issue of implementation.

Health promotion in action

Parry Langdon et al. (2003) present two examples of evaluation of programmes seeking to reduce smoking in schools. Both sought to control the 'captive communities' in the intervention schools, using quantitative methods to measure the effectiveness of the programmes in reducing the prevalence of smoking (the outcome). They both also incorporated process evaluation. The methods used were face-to-face semi-structured interviews with pupils and teachers, focus groups, workshops and questionnaires. The authors value this mixed-methods approach because it allows different stakeholders to express their views about how the intervention was received in the schools. Differing stakeholder groups could interpret success differently; evaluating the process (with a large amount of qualitative data) gave insight into why the interventions did or did not work. The authors also planned to evaluate the impact that the interventions might have had on the curriculum and school policies.

It would seem most appropriate for those seeking to carry out EBHP to draw on both outcome and process evaluation in order to benefit from the richest and widest evidence around. This is not only to ascertain what interventions were successful in meeting their outcomes, but what contextual factors might have influenced the success of the intervention. Answers to these questions prove to be extremely valuable to health promoters wishing to make evidence based decisions in their own practice.

Additional point

One interesting approach to measuring outcomes is to use community defined indicators. These can be used to describe the current state of health, education, environmental quality or access to local services and are, therefore, related to broad factors that influence health – and those factors that are usually prioritized by the local communities. Health promotion interventions could tackle a variety of these issues, and compare the indicators before and after the intervention. Examples given by MacGillivray et al. (1998) include:

- Kilometres of dedicated cycle routes
- Road casualties
- Local air pollution
- Number of adult residents in training or education
- Decay in children's teeth
- Perception of personal safety at night
- Number of allotments in use
- Percentage of tree cover
- Participation in decision-making

> ### Tutorial brief 6.2
>
> What are the pros and cons of using community indicators rather than traditional epidemiological data (such as teenage pregnancy rates) as evidence of the success or otherwise of a health promotion intervention?

A widescreen approach

Health promotion is increasingly concerned with issues beyond individual behaviour-change, focusing on socio-environmental factors and consideration of power, equity and 'community' (see Chapter 1). Labonte and Robertson (1996: 433) put it that:

> Empowerment is a very different phenomenon than serum cholesterol ... To investigate empowerment using a research paradigm appropriate to an investigation of serum cholesterol, as is often the case in health promotion research, is to commit a fundamental error.

As health promotion practice tackles these wider issues, so should our view of what constitutes evidence and what is appropriate to form the evidence base of health promotion. Our worldview needs to become more 'widescreen'. Taking on board these ideas, health promotion is gradually moving to a pluralistic approach to building its evidence base, drawing on a range of methods to inform practice and generate evidence. Petticrew and Roberts (2003) suggest that qualitative research methods should be considered along with quantitative methods in a typology (classification by type), rather than a hierarchy. This is dependant, though, on the questions being asked. Methodologically speaking, a 'horses for courses' approach would be most realistic and practical. This is a result of an approach, incorporating pragmatism, that seeks to improve services or empower people, or is based on the understanding that evidence based health promotion needs to draw on a range of evidence from other disciplines (McQueen 2001). Since its work is often multi-sectoral in nature, so nurses and other health care practitioners should be aware of evidence from a variety of fields. However, evidence based practice information might be difficult to interpret without sector-specific knowledge (Armstrong et al. 2006). For example, nurses might find evidence from adult education harder to interpret than evidence from a health discipline.

Evidence based health promotion in practice

Once a practitioner has decided that they wish to implement a health promotion intervention that is evidence based, what process do they need to go through?

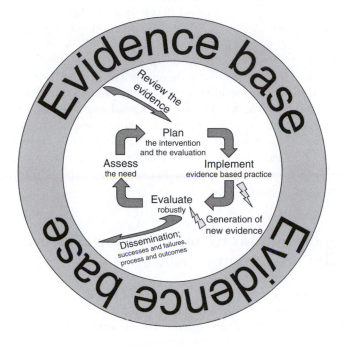

Figure 6.2 Health promotion in the context of the evidence base

Figure 6.2 sets out the systematic process of health promotion (as discussed in Chapter 4), and places it in context of the evidence base.

Once the health promoter has assessed the need for a health promotion intervention, a review should be conducted of the available evidence on that intervention. This, in itself, is a process, involving finding the evidence, using cross-disciplinary searches and then critically appraising the relevance of each piece of evidence. The nurse should consider relevance to the local situation and also to local organizational factors. Wang et al. (2005) discuss interventions in terms of *applicability* (where the process could be transferred to another setting) and *transferability* (whether the effectiveness or outcomes could be achievable in another setting). Once again, the context is key to the successful implementation of health promotion interventions: 'external evidence can inform, but can never replace, the expertise of individual practitioners' (Tang et al. 2003: 482), and research evidence will always need to be adapted to fit local circumstances (Nutbeam 1996). Once the evidence has been appraised, the intervention can be implemented, after any necessary resources have been negotiated. Figure 6.2 indicates that the planning stage should also include the planning of any evaluation methods. It is important not to leave evaluation planning until towards the end of a health promotion activity (see Chapter 4). During the implementation and evaluation stages of the systematic process of health promotion, new evidence can be generated as appropriate research or evaluation methodologies are applied (Rychetnik and Wise 2004).

New evidence generated as part of the health promotion intervention is useful for the practitioner in demonstrating the effectiveness and success, or otherwise, of their programme. However, it is important that this evidence is disseminated to the wider community of health promoters, thereby enhancing the overall evidence base of health promotion. The elements that affected the process, as well as the outcomes, should be shared so that others can learn. McDonald and Veihbeck (2007) advocate the development of 'communities of practice', where researchers and practitioners work together and share information on a particular problem or issue. McDonald and Veihbeck (2007: 142) assert that: 'The focus of the community is not only on *sharing* "best" practices but also on *creating* knowledge and resources to advance the practice or issue of interest.'

Barriers and solutions to implementing evidence based health promotion

So far, this chapter has discussed the importance of EBHP, while acknowledging the tensions between research and practice and the different paradigms, leading to some methodologies being favoured over others. The context of the evidence base within the structured process of health promotion has been discussed, and the need for a 'widescreen' view of evidence based practice has been called for. However, several authors have examined the use of evidence by a variety of health professionals and found that there are several barriers to implementing evidence based practice (for example, James et al. 2007 – health promoters; Metcalfe et al. 2001 – professions allied to medicine, and Gerrish et al. 2007 and Thompson et al. 2005 – nurses). These barriers include:

- A lack of time for staff to access evidence
- Lack of access to databases
- Perceived lack of skills in searching for evidence
- Team or organizational reluctance to change
- Lack of priority given to reading research
- Problems with the presentation of evidence – such as:
  - ○ Implications for practice not clear
  - ○ Evidence not perceived as relevant
  - ○ Evidence not presented in an understandable manner
  - ○ Evidence too focused on the biomedical model

However, Armstrong et al. (2007) warn that, even when 'evidence-based health promotion resources' were produced and circulated in Victoria, Australia, this information alone was unlikely to be a catalyst for change. They suggest that practitioner engagement and knowledge-management processes are required.

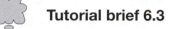 **Tutorial brief 6.3**

Given the barriers in implementing evidence based health promotion already identified, what solutions can you suggest to overcome these?

Possible solutions could include additional development in searching and critical appraisal skills through continuing professional development and developing part-nerships with academics and researchers (South and Tilford 2000). These approaches could support practitioners in developing methodologically robust approaches to evidence generation and a renewed emphasis that decision-making should be evidence based – which might come about through improved dialogue between practitioners, researchers and managers. Publications in some journals are now including a table giving an overview of 'what we know already' and 'what this paper adds', which could help practitioners assess the relevance of the paper. 'Communi-ties of learning' (McDonald and Viehbeck 2007) could support the design of research projects or evaluation, along with supporting staff to disseminate their findings. This, in turn, could address the lack of practice based evidence available to nurses and the wider community of health promotion practitioners.

Conclusion

Since health promotion owes as much to social science as it does to medicine, then evidence based health promotion practice owes as much to qualitative approaches as it does to quantitative approaches. In order for nurses and other health profes-sionals to deliver EBHP, they must be able to draw widely on evidence from a range of disciplines and be aware of the pitfalls of limiting their evidence base to narrow definitions of evidence. A 'wide screen view' is required, since health promotion often entails complex interventions that are context-specific. The model presented in this chapter (Figure 6.2) demonstrates the relationship between systematic process of health promotion and the health promotion evidence base, requiring the appraisal of evidence to inform practice and, equally importantly, the dissemination of findings (through evaluation of process and outcome) to inform and build the evidence base for health promotion.

Additional resources

Cochrane collaboration. Systematic reviews on health care. Available online at www.cochrane.org
EPPI Centre. An online evidence library, including a section containing systematic reviews on health promotion topics. Available online at http://eppi.ioe.ac.uk/cms/Default.aspx?tabid=56
International Union for health promotion and education. Some useful resources, including access to 'Promotion and Education'. Available online at http://www.iuhpe.org/index.html

National Library for Health (NLH). Available online at www.library.nhs.uk
National Institute for Health and Clinical Excellence. Available online at http://www.nice.org.uk/
    guidance/
NHS Centre for Reviews and Dissemination, University of York. Available online at www.york.ac.uk/
    onst/crd/
The Community Guide. Evidence based recommendations for programmes and policies to promote
    population health. Available online at http://www.thecommunityguide.org/
WHO health promotion site. Available online at http://www.who.int/healthpromotion/en/

References

Armstrong, R., Doyle, J., Lamb, C. and Waters, E. (2006) 'Multi-sectoral Health Promotion and Public
    Health: The Role of Evidence', *Journal of Public Health*, 28(2): 168–72.
Armstrong, R., Waters, E., Crockett, B. and Keleher, H. (2007) 'The Nature of Evidence Resources and
    Knowledge Translation for Health Promotion Practitioners', *Health Promotion International*, 22(3):
    254–60.
Baum, F. (1995) 'Researching Public Health: Beyond The Qualitative–Quantitative Methodological
    Debate', *Social Science and Medicine*, 40(4): 459–68.
Bisset, S., Cargo, M., Delormier, T., Macaulay, A.C. and Potvin, L. (2004) 'Legitimizing Diabetes as a
    Community Health Issue: A Case Analysis of an Aboriginal Community in Canada', *Health Promotion
    International*, 19(3): 317–26.
Bowling, A. (2002) *Research Methods in Health: Investigating Health and Health Services*, 2nd edn
    (Milton Keynes: Open University Press).
Britton, A., Thorogood, M., Coombes, Y., Lewando-Hundt, G., Sheldon, T.A. Sowden, A.J. and Lister-
    Sharp, D. (1998) 'Search for Evidence of Effective Health Promotion', *BMJ*, 316: 703.
Chen, M., Liou, Y. and Wu, J. (2008) 'The Relationship between TV/Computer Time and Adolescents'
    Health Promoting Behaviour: A Secondary Data Analysis', *Journal of Nursing Research*, 16(1):
    75–84.
Coote, A., Allen, J. and Woodhead, D. (2004) *Finding Out What Works: Building Knowledge
    About Complex Community-Based Initiatives* (London: Kings Fund). Available online at www.
    kingsfund.org
Cornwall, A. (1996) 'Towards Participatory Practice: Participatory Rural Appraisal (PRA) and the
    Participatory Process', in De Koning, K. and Martin, M. (eds), *Participatory Research in Health: Issues
    and Experiences* (London: Zed Books).
Daly, J., Willis, R., Small, K., Green, J., Welch, N., Keal, M. and Hughes, E. (2007) 'A Hierarchy of
    Evidence for Assessing Qualitative Health Research', *Journal of Clinical Epidemiology*, 60: 43–9.
Denzin, N.K. (1989) *The Research Act: A Theoretical Introduction to Sociological Methods*, 3rd edn
    (New Jersey: Prentice Hall).
DoH (2004) *Choosing Health: Making Healthy Choices Easier* (London: TSO).
DoH (2006) *Our Health, Our Care, Our Say: A New Direction For Community Services* (London: TSO).
El Ansari, W. (2005) 'Collaborative Research Partnerships with Disadvantaged Communities: Challenges
    and Potential Solutions', *Public Health*, 119(9): 758–70.
Elliott, H. and Popay, J. (2000) 'How Are Policy Makers Using Evidence? Models of Research Utilisation
    and Local NHS Policy Making', *Journal of Epidemiology and Community Health*, 54: 461–8.
Evans, D. (2003) 'Hierarchy of Evidence: A Framework for Ranking Evidence Evaluating Healthcare
    Interventions', *Journal of Clinical Nursing*, 12(1): 77–84.
Feuerstein, M.T. (1986) *Partners in Evaluation: Evaluating Development and Community Programmes
    with Participants* (London: Macmillan/TALC).
Freire, P. (1972) *Pedagogy of the Oppressed* (London: Penguin).
Gerrish, K., Ashworth, P., Lacey, A, Bailey, J., Cooke, J., Kendall, S. and McNeilly, E. (2007) 'Factors
    Influencing the Development of Evidence-based Practice: A Research Tool', *Journal of Advanced
    Nursing*, 57(3): 328–38.

Howes, F., Doyle, J., Jackson, N. and Waters, E. (2004) 'Evidence-based Public Health: The Importance of Finding "Difficult To Locate" Public Health and Health Promotion Intervention Studies for Systematic Reviews', *Journal of Public Health*, 26(1): 101–4.

Inchley, J., Muldoon, J. and Currie, C. (2006) 'Becoming a Health Promoting School: Evaluating the Process of Effective Implementation in Scotland', *Health Promotion International*, 22(1): 65–71.

Jackson, N. and Waters, E. (2005) 'Criteria for the Systematic Review of Health Promotion and Public Health Interventions', *Health Promotion International*, 20(4): 367–74.

James, E.L., Fraiser, C., Anderson, K. and Judd, F. (2007) 'Use of Research by the Australian Health Promotion Workforce', *Health Education Research*, 22(4): 576–87.

Jamieson, L.M., Parker, E.J. and Richards, L. (2007) 'Using Qualitative Methodology to Inform an Indigenous-owned Oral Health Promotion Initiative in Australia', *Health Promotion International*, 23(1): 52–9.

Katainen, A. (2006) 'Challenging the Imperative of Health? Smoking and Justifications of Risk-taking', *Critical Public Health*, 16(4): 295–305.

Labonte, R., Feather, J. and Hills, M. (1999) 'A Story/Dialogue Method for Health Promotion Knowledge Development and Evaluation', *Health Education Research*, 14(1): 39–50.

Labonte, R. and Robertson, A. (1996) 'Delivering the Goods, Showing Our Stuff: The Case for a Constructivist Paradigm for Health Promotion Research and Practice', *Health Education Quarterly*, 23: 431–47.

Learmonth, A.M. (2000) 'Utilizing Research in Practice and Generating Evidence from Practice', *Health Education Research*, 15(6): 743–56.

Learmonth, A.M. and Watson, N.J. (1999) 'Constructing Evidence-based Health Promotion: Perspectives from the Field', *Critical Public Health*, 9(4): 317–33.

MacGillivray, A., Weston, C. and Unsworth, C. (1998) *Communities Count: A Step By Step Guide To Community Sustainability Indicators* (London: New Economics Foundation).

Macnee, C.L. and McCabe, S. (2008) *Understanding Nursing Research: Reading and Using Research in Evidence-based Practice*, 2nd edn (Philadelphia: Lippincott Williams & Wilkins).

McDonald, P.W. and Viehback, S. (2007) 'From Evidence-based Practice Making to Practice-based Evidence Making: Creating Communities of (Research) and Practice, *Health Promotion Practice*, 8(20): 140–4.

McQueen, D.V. (2001) 'Strengthening the Evidence Base for Health Promotion', *Health Promotion International*, 16(3): 261–8.

McVicar, M. (1999) 'Integrating Research into Nursing Practice', in Perkins, E.R., Simnet, I. and Wright, L. (eds), *Evidence-based Health Promotion* (Chichester: Wiley).

Meyer, J. (2000) 'Using Qualitative Methods in Health Related Action Research', *BMJ*, 320: 178–81.

Metcalfe, C., Lewin, R., Wishes, S., Bannigan, K. and Klaber Moffett, J. (2001) 'Barriers to Implementing the Evidence Base in Four NHS Therapies', *Physiotherapy*, 87(8): 433–41.

NICE (2008) *Community Engagement to Improve Health*, NICE Public Health Guidance (London, NICE).

Nutbeam, D. (1996) 'Achieving "Best Practice" in Health Promotion: Improving the Fit between Research and Practice', *Health Education Research*, 11(3): 317–26.

Nutbeam, D. (2000) 'Health Promotion Effectiveness – The Questions To Be Answered', in International Union for Health Promotion and Education (IUHPE), *The Evidence of Health Promotion Effectiveness: Shaping Public Health in a New Europe*, Part 2 (Luxembourg: IUHPE).

Nutbeam, D., MacAskill, P and Smith, C. (1993) 'Evaluation of Two Schools Smoking Education Programmes under Normal Classroom Conditions, *BMJ*, 306: 102–7.

O'Dwyer, L.A., Baum, F., Kavanagh, A. and Macdougall, C. (2007) 'Do Area-based Interventions to Reduce Health Inequalities Work? A Systematic Review of Evidence', *Critical Public Health*, 17(4): 317–35.

Parry Langdon, N., Bloor, M., Audrey, S. and Holliday, J. (2003) 'Process Evaluation of Health Promotion Interventions', *Policy & Politics*, 31(2): 207–16.

Perkins, E., Simnett, I. and Wright, L. (1999) *Evidence-Based Health Promotion* (Chichester: Wiley).

Petticrew, M. and Roberts, H. (2003) Evidence, Hierarchies, and Typologies: Horses for Courses', *Journal of Epidemiology and Community Health*, 57: 527–9.

Polit, D.F. and Beck, C.T. (2006) *Essentials of Nursing Research: Methods, Appraisal, and Utilization*, 6th edn (Philadelphia: Lippincott Williams & Wilkins).

Popay, J. and Williams, G. (1996) 'Public Health Research and Lay Knowledge', *Social Science and Medicine*, 42(5): 759–68.

Rada, J., Ratima, M. and Howden-Chapman, P. (1999) 'Evidence-based Purchasing of Health Promotion: Methodology for Reviewing Evidence', *Health Promotion International*, 14: 177–87.

Ravesloot, C.H, Seekins, T., Cahill, T. and Lindgren, S. (2007) 'Health Promotion for People with Disabilities: Development and Evaluation of The Living Well with a Disability Programme', *Health Education Research*, 22(4): 522–31.

Rhodes, S., Foley, K., Zometa, C. and Bloom F. (2007) 'Lay Health Advisor Interventions among Hispanics/Latinos: A Qualitative Systematic Review', *American Journal of Preventive Medicine*, 33(5): 418–27.

Rosen, L., Manor, O., Engelhard, D. and Zucker, D. (2006) 'In Defence of the Randomized Controlled Trial for Health Promotion Research', *American Journal of Public Health*, 96: 1181–6.

Rychetnik, L. and Wise, M. (2004) 'Advocating Evidence-based Health Promotion: Reflections and a Way Forward', *Health Promotion International*, 19(2): 247–57.

Rycroft-Malone, J., Seers, K., Titchin, A., Harvey, G., Kitson, A. and McCormack, B. (2004) 'What Counts as Evidence in Evidence-based Practice?', *Journal of Advanced Nursing*, 47(1): 81–90.

Sackett, D., Rosenberg, W., Gray, J., Haynes, B. and Richardson, S. (1996) 'Evidence-based Medicine: What It Is and What It Isn't', *BMJ*, 312: 71–2.

Scott, D., Rhodes, S.D., Long Foley, K., Zometa, C.S. and Bloom, F.R. (2007) 'Lay Health Advisor Interventions among Hispanics/Latinos: A Qualitative Systematic Review', *American Journal of Preventive Medicine*, 33(5): 418–27.

Seedhouse, D. (1996) *Health Promotion: Philosophy, Prejudice and Practice* (Chichester: Wiley).

Smith, B.J., Tang K.C. and Nutbeam, D. (2006) 'WHO Health Promotion Glossary: New Terms', *Health Promotion International* (Oxford: Oxford University Press).

South, J. and Tilford, S. (2000) 'Perceptions of Research and Evaluation in Health Promotion Practice and Influences on Activity', *Health Education Research*, 15: 729–41.

Speller, V., Learmonth, A. and Harrison, D. (1997) 'The Search for Evidence of Effective Health Promotion', *BMJ*, 315: 361–3.

Springett, J., Owens, C. and Callaghan, J. (2007) 'The Challenge of Combining "Lay" Knowledge With "Evidence-based" Practice in Health Promotion: Fag Ends Smoking Cessation Service', *Critical Public Health*, 17(3): 243–56.

Stephenson, J.M., Strange, V., Forrest, S., Oakley, A., Copas, A., Allen, E., Babiker, A., Black, S., Ali, M., Monteiro, H. and Johnson, A.M. (2004) 'Pupil-led Sex Education in England (RIPPLE Study): Cluster-randomised Intervention Trial', *Lancet*, 364: 338–46.

Stewart-Brown, S. (2001) 'Evaluating Health Promotion in Schools: Reflections', in Rootman, I., Hyndman, B. and McQueen, D.V. (eds), 'Evaluation in Health Promotion. Principles and Perspectives', WHO Regional Publications European Series, 92 (Copenhagen: WHO, Regional Office for Europe).

Tang, K.C., Ehsani, J.P. and McQueen, D.V. (2003) 'Evidence Based Health Promotion: Recollections, Reflections, and Reconsiderations', *Journal of Epidemiology and Community Health*, 57(11): 841–3.

Thomas, R. and Perera, R. (2006) 'School-based Programmes for Preventing Smoking', *Cochrane Database of Systematic Reviews*, 3, art. no.: CD001293.

Thompson, C., McCaughan, D., Cullum, N., Sheldon, T. and Raynor, P. (2005) 'Barriers to Evidence-based Practice in Primary Care Nursing – Why Viewing Decision-making as Context Is Helpful', *Journal of Advanced Nursing*, 52(4): 432–44.

Tilford, S. (2000) 'Editorial: Evidence-based Health Promotion', *Health Education Research*, 15(6): 659–63.

Torgerson, C.J. (2006) 'Publication Bias: The Achilles' Heel of Systematic Reviews?', *British Journal of Educational Studies*, 54(1): 89–102.

Wang, S., Moss, J.R. and Hiller, J.E. (2005) 'Applicability and Transferability of Interventions in Evidence-based Public Health', *Health Promotion International*, 21(1): 76–83.

Whitehead, D. (2003) 'Evaluating Health Promotion: A Model for Nursing Practice', *Journal of Advanced Nursing*, 41(5): 490–8.

Whitehead, D. and Elliot, D. (2007) 'Mixed Methods Research', in Schneider, Z., Whitehead, D., Elliott, D., LoBiondo-Wood, G. and Haber, J., *Nursing and Midwifery Research: Methods and Appraisal for Evidence-based Practice*, 3rd edn (Sydney, Australia: Elsevier/Mosby): 248–67.

WHO (no date) 'Global Programme on Health Promotion Effectiveness' (GPHPE). Available online at http://www.who.int/healthpromotion/areas/gphpe/en/index.html

WHO (1986) *Ottawa Charter for Health Promotion*, An International Conference on Health Promotion. The Move Towards a New Public Health, 17–21 November, Ottawa, Canada.

WHO (1997) 'The Jakarta Declaration on Leading Health Promotion into the 21st Century', *Health Promotion International*, 12: 261–26.

WHO (1998a) *Health Promotion Evaluation: Recommendations to Policy Holders*, Report of the WHO European Working Group on Health Promotion (Copenhagen: WHO).

WHO (1998b) *Health Promotion Glossary* (Geneva: WHO).

WHO (2007) 'Health Evidence Network' (HEN). Available at http://www.euro.who.int/HEN/RelatedSites/20060529_17

Wilhelmsson, S. and Lindberg, M. (2007) *International Journal of Nursing Practice*, 13: 254–66.

Wimbush, E. and Watson J. (2000) 'An Evaluation Framework for Health Promotion: Theory, Quality and Effectiveness', *Evaluation*, 6: 301–21.

CHAPTER 7

Health Promotion: Politics, Policy and Ethics

Rod Thomson

Objectives

By the end of this chapter you should be able to:

- Identify what is meant by ethics in relation to health promotion and examine examples of ethical challenges in health promotion practice
- Identify what is meant by politics in relation to health promotion and examine examples of political challenges in health promotion practice
- Consider strategies for conducting health promotion within ethical and political constraints and frameworks
- Examine the processes by which health policy underpins health promotion activity

Key terms

- Ethics
- Harm reduction
- Health inequalities
- Policy
- Politics
- Society

Introduction

To paraphrase an American saying, 'Health promotion is like motherhood or apple pie'. In other words, it is a subject that most people would endorse as a positive idea. However, as with the concept of motherhood and the recipe for apple pie, behind the high level consensus there is wide scope for a variety of views about what constitutes a good mother, a good apple pie and, of course, 'good' health promotion.

The concept of health promotion is something that most nurses would support yet, when it comes to applying it to everyday practice, this consensus begins to fragment (see the earlier chapters of this book). This particular chapter focuses on the ethical and political factors that might influence the way in which health promotion is implemented. This chapter will draw on examples from around the globe that illustrate how public and political opinion can have positive and negative impacts on health promotion programmes. Examples from the field of HIV/AIDS prevention (covered also in Chapter 8) will be utilized as, in the last twenty years or so, this area of health care has touched every corner of the globe. The HIV/AIDS pandemic has been identified by the World Health Organization (WHO) as one of the greatest health challenges ever to the Earth's population. As one of the main methods of transmission of the HIV virus is sexual intercourse, an action arguably essential for the continuation of humankind, this area of health promotion has implications for everyone on the planet. However, as this chapter intends to illustrate, while there is broad consensus about the need to prevent the spread of HIV, the approaches taken across the globe vary significantly. In some cases, such variation might be attributed to the relative affluence of a country and its ability to deploy resources towards tackling the problem. In other cases, the political context within the country and the prevailing religious/cultural background profoundly affect courses of health action. Factors that appear to influence health promotion programmes adversely, in relation to HIV prevention, are often linked to drugs misuse and perceived sexual deviancy or promiscuity. This chapter will consider these topics to highlight how approaches to health promotion have been influenced across the globe as well as their ethical, political and policy implication and, consequently, their implications for nursing practice.

The context of HIV/AIDS in relation to health promotion

It could be argued that most nurses will not be involved in any health promotion activity related to HIV/AIDS prevention. If that is the case, why should it be used as the basis of this chapter? For nurses working in acute hospitals or with particular sections of the population, such as children or older people, the relevance of this issue to their usual field of practice might seem remote. Yet, as examples will illustrate, many children will have their first sexual experiences before the age of consent. Therefore, for nurses working with school-age children, sex health and relationship education will be a key area of their health promotion practice. In Western Europe, North America and Australasia, health services are treating patients whose substance misusing careers began in the 1960s. Those individuals in their teens and twenties back then are now in their sixties and seventies. For some of these individuals, their use of drugs such as cannabis and methadone continues and, therefore, the risk of drug related harm does so too. Finally, while diseases such as cholera, dysentery and malaria cause significant levels of death and disease across the world, in general they tend to affect fewer countries when compared with HIV/AIDS. In view of their global reach and impact, HIV and AIDS issues can be argued as a good starting point to consider the ethical and political factors that might influence health promotion strategy. As the United Nations (UN) highlighted in their *Millennium Goals* statement, the extent of the pandemic is such to merit a concerted health promotion and harm reduction effort across the world. They (UN 2001) state:

In June 2001, Heads of State and Representatives of Governments met at the United Nations General Assembly Special Session dedicated to HIV/AIDS. The meeting was a major milestone in the AIDS response. It was recognized that the AIDS epidemic had caused untold suffering and death worldwide. The UN Special Session also served to remind the world that there was hope. With sufficient will and resources, communities and countries could change the epidemic's deadly course. The theme global crisis requiring global action served to underline the need for urgent attention. At the meeting, Heads of State and Representatives of Governments issued the Declaration of Commitment on HIV/AIDS. The Declaration remains a powerful tool that is helping to guide and secure action, commitment, support and resources for the AIDS response.

Ethics: what it is and why is it important to health promotion

Ethics and ethical behaviour are seen as important components of health care. One of Florence Nightingale's core principles was that we 'should do the sick no harm'. The UK's Nursing and Midwifery Council's (NMC) Code, which sets the standards of conduct, performance and ethics for nurses and midwives, also highlights the fundamental premise that nurses must make the care of people their first concern, treating them as individuals and respecting their dignity (NMC 2008). The code highlights a number of key themes that are directly related to ethical behaviour by the profession. For example, it states that: The people in your care must be able to trust you with their health and Wellbeing, and 'You must be open and hones, act with integrity and uphold the reputation of your profession.'

Similar codes of ethics/conduct can be found across the globe, particularly in Western societies. The additional resources section at the end of this chapter contains details of the websites for some of these nursing bodies. Nurses in Taiwan conducted a major review of their code of ethics in 2006 (Chiou-Fen Lin 2007). Within their new code were 27 fundamental principles, of which those in the following list are worthy of note in relation to political and policy responsibilities. They are firmly grounded within the ethos of health promotion theory and practice. They are:

- Nurses have responsibilities of health promotion, disease prevention, health restoration and suffering relief to clients. (1)
- Nurses shall use resources equally and will not provide clients with different services because of their own preferences or clients socioeconomic status. (4)

- Nurses shall actively participate in activities that will promote the health of the general public and educate people to increase their knowledge and ability of health maintenance. (18)
- Nurses shall be concerned about the social, economic, environmental, and political factors that would affect health, and aggressively participate in advocating and promoting related policies according to their own specialities. (19)

Note: The numbers at the end of each line relate to the numbering system used by the Taiwanese Ethical Code of Conduct.

While the notion that nurses have a responsibility for conducting health promotion, disease prevention and health restoration will come as no surprise to most people, item 4 of the Taiwanese Ethical Code of Conduct might be an unexpected addition. For Taiwanese nurses, it seems that it is not enough to be concerned about the social, economic, environmental and political factors that might affect health. The new Ethical Code of Conduct encourages them to participate aggressively in advocating and promoting related policies that will enhance the health and well-being of their clients.

Trevor Clay, a former general secretary of the Royal College of Nursing (UK) and a former member of the Board of Directors of the International Council of Nurses (ICN), considered the ethical dilemmas facing nurses in his book *Nurses: Power and Politics* (Clay 1987). He believed that one of the great strengths of the nursing profession – its concentration on the personal and individual needs of the patient – was also the profession's greatest weakness. This focus, he argued, caused nurses to leave ethical issues to others – often the medical and legal professions – rather than assert their own views based on the unique relationship nurses have with the patients and communities in their care. Clay (1987) argued that nurses are:

required to deny their own feelings and the needs to create confidence and calm in others. Too many nurses take that suppression of their individual feeling on a daily basis into political life. Nursing is perhaps the most unassertive profession in the UK, yet more than ever, we need collectively to look beyond immediate problems and preoccupations to see the forces that are active around us and to tackle them.

Twenty years on, the Taiwanese Ethical Code of Conduct provides an example of how the profession recognizes that it has a duty to speak and act assertively in order to secure the health and well-being of the patients and communities it serves. Many nurses are beginning to realize this as part of their health promotion role.

Human rights are seen as the core of all nursing practice. The ICN states that:

Nurses have an obligation to safeguard and actively promote people's health rights at all times and in all places ... Nurses deal with human rights daily, in all aspects of their professional as such, they might be pressured to apply their knowledge and skills in ways that are detrimental to patients and others. Furthermore nurses are increasingly facing complex human rights issues, arising from conflict situations within jurisdictions, political upheaval and wars.

The British Medical Association (BMA) sets out similar principles on its website for its members in relation to ethical behaviour and human rights (BMA 2008). They can be found at www.bma.org.uk/ap.nsf/Content/MedProfhumanRights-Recommendations

While the focus of these human rights statements was, and is, clinical treatment, this ethical underpinning of practice applies directly to health promotion activity, too. Other chapters of this book have set out what health promotion is and the methods by which it can be carried out; this chapter will set aside the need to explain these topics. Instead, it will concentrate on the practical aspects of the impacts of ethics on the promotion of health and well-being of individuals, communities and societies.

Ethics related to the well-being of individuals, communities and societies

In general terms, most societies acknowledge the concept of self-determination or free will for their citizens, or the right to choose the way of life each individual will follow. Some exceptions will be made as to which citizens can exercise free will. For example, children, prisoners and individuals with mental health problems might have restrictions on the choices they can make for themselves. However, the exercise of free will might also mean that individuals can make a choice that will place them at risk of short- or long- term injury – or even death. For example boxers, mountain climbers and rugby players place themselves at risk each time they train or take part in their chosen sport. Though there are some sections of society that would wish to ban boxing or prevent children from playing rugby, most people would not challenge an individual's right to play their sport of choice. However, as the nurses who might have to treat such patients, we might have personal views about the risks that have been taken that adversely affect our practice and resources.

Rothstein and Phuong (2007) examined the ethical attitudes of the Institutional Board members in 27 hospitals across 12 US states. While their study focused on the members' attitudes to the ethical issues in human subject research, it highlighted the contrasts between the physicians and unaffiliated members – and the nurses on these boards. They concluded that:

> Nurses had the greatest concern with ethical issues of the major groups that serve on IRBs (Institutional Review Boards) but had little influence on IRB deliberations. Their lack of influence might be related to the presence of only one nurse among the 10 members of the average IRB.

As nurses are the largest group of professionals providing health care, and have the greatest contact with patients, such a disparity emphasizes the need for nurses to be more assertive in promoting and advocating for the health of their patients (see Chapter 1).

Additional point

In the field of drug misuse treatment, nurses are often at the cutting edge of health promotion and treatment, but the medical profession in general – and psychiatrists in particular – often have greater influence on the development of policy and research.

Drug misuse evokes a greater level of condemnation from a broader section of society than activities such as boxing. This is perhaps due to the scale of drug misuse worldwide. Dr Ian Oliver, an independent consultant to the United Nations Drug Control Programme, estimated that around 200 million people use illicit drugs. While marijuana/cannabis was identified as the most commonly used drug, with an estimated 160 million users worldwide, there are also around 16 million opiate users and 14 million cocaine users (Oliver 2006) Drugs misuse can cause a variety of short- and long-term health problems. It is also responsible for the deaths of many drug users through overdose, or from blood-borne viruses such as HIV/AIDS and a range of hepatitis related disorders. Later in this chapter we will consider some of the challenges for nurses involved in health promotion with drug users.

Additional point

The UK's Royal College of Nursing has an ethics forum as one of its specialist sub-groups. Membership is free to RCN members. The forum acts as a focus for consideration of ethical matters related to nursing. In addition, the forum works with other professional and patients representative organizations on cross-cutting ethical issues.

Summary point

Nursing representative bodies across the globe recognize that nurses must conduct their professional practice within an ethical framework that recognizes the human rights of the individuals and communities they provide care for, including health promotion activities. Ethics can be seen as a code of behaviour or a moral framework that can be used by nurses to guide their actions when working with areas of human activity that are contentious or illegal.

Politics: What is it and why is it important to health promotion?

Politics can be described as the art and science of government, or:

> The activities associated with governing a country or area, and the political relations between states or a particular set of political beliefs or principles, or activities aimed at gaining power within an organization. (Oxford English Dictionary 2002)

Across the globe, governments fund some form of health care for their citizens. This can vary from minimal levels of state support for emergency care, such as the USA, to the universal provision of almost all aspects of health care – for example, Denmark and the UK. Spread across this continuum is a wide variety of models in which citizens can access some level of state support, with those remaining aspects of health care being paid directly by the citizen or through some form of insurance scheme. The basis for these diverse systems can be attributed to political ideology on health services.

Within democratic societies, political parties seek the support of the electorate for the policies they wish to make into legislation. The factors that will influence the electorate to support the policies of a political party are complex. Some factors will be very pragmatic – such as how much taxation voters will have to pay to support a particular set of policies and the benefits they will receive in return. Other factors will be influenced by less tangible issues, and will reflect the belief system that underpins the ideals and aspirations of the same individuals. Religious belief, cultural upbringing and education might influence how individuals view the society in which they live and, in turn, affect their views about the political parties that seek their votes.

To be voted into government, a political party must win the popular approval of its electorate. In view of this necessity, political parties are likely to tailor their political philosophy to incorporate populous measures into their election manifestos and policies. Such necessities have an effect on public health policy and the delivery of health promotion programmes. This particularly applies to more controversial areas of public health promotion such as HIV/AIDS, drug misuse and sexual health. These topics will be used in this chapter to illustrate the influence politics can have on health promotion practice.

One of the key driving forces in politics is the desire to change the way a community is run. Whether that community is a town, a city, a region or a country, the principle is the same – 'politicians' seek control of community resources in order to shape a community in line with their views. It is this control of resources that affects health promotion practitioners, and the policies and practices they wish to enact. Clay (1987) believed that nurses isolated themselves from the political process as a profession; hence his stated objective to bring nurses and nursing more openly into politics:

> It is only by fighting and winning battles over resources, organization and policy in the public arena that we can avoid those conflicts intruding into the private and personal relationships that individual nurses must have with the people they serve.

Clay's successor, Dr Peter Carter, also emphasized the scale of the challenge faced by nurses in the UK to achieve and maintain effective engagement at all levels of the political process. He argued that most health related policy is developed without significant input from nurses (Snow 2009). Whitehead (2003) also highlighted the challenges facing the profession across the globe in articulating its expertise to policy-makers and persuading governments to listen to the views of nurses. Within the UK, for instance, such views have led to the development of specific political leadership programmes for nurses interested in being politically active. This programme can be accessed at: www.rcn.org.uk/learningzone

It should be recognized, though, that nurses and other health practitioners are not passive objects being tossed back and forth by the changing winds of political fortune. Nurses, in particular, have the ability to influence political and public opinion. In part, this is due to their role as the largest group of professional carers in the health care systems of most countries. It is also due to their voting power in democratic countries. Properly harnessed nurses, and their families and friends, represent significant numbers of voters in every electoral area and, as such, are a pressure group no politician or government can ignore. However, although there have been more and more recent examples of nurses exercising their political 'muscle' throughout the world, this has generally related to campaigns for pay and conditions. To campaign for health promotion, nurses must be able to marshal the evidence to demonstrate why they wish to take a particular course of health promotion action and what it will achieve. Nurses and other health practitioners must also be able to demonstrate a level of political awareness and the skill to enable them to work effectively within the setting within which they work (Drucker 1999).

Drucker (1999) reviewed a quarter century of political conflict in the USA regarding national drug policy, and demonstrated how the weight of evidence in favour of 'harm reduction' has struggled to influence national government. He argued that America had lost its 'war on drugs' and that there was a need for significant change. He stated:

> These are not-so-early warning signs of a great American failure – not only in drug policy but also in our native capacity for creative, compassionate, and above all open discourse about issues vital to our well-being. It is time that we move beyond this drug fundamentalism and abandon our unhappy history of prohibition for more humane and pragmatic policies that protect public health and support our democratic values.

In the recent US presidential campaign, American nurses campaigned strongly in favour of Barak Obama. It will be interesting to see whether they will use the political influence gained from the election of President Obama to lobby for the changes that Drucker and his organization have advocated.

Summary point

While there are different systems of government across the world, their common point is that an aim of each system is to control and utilize the resources of a community to achieve the goals of each government.

Nurses across the globe must work within these systems and use the mechanisms open to them to influence governmental policy development and use of resources if they are to maximize their ability to promote the health and well-being of the individuals and communities they serve. An understanding of the political system at local and national level in the country in which a nurse lives and works is an important basis for advocating effectively on behalf of the health of the patients she/he serves.

The context of the HIV/AIDS pandemic

The global pandemic of HIV/AIDS is perhaps one of the best examples of the challenges facing public health and health promotion in the world today. In the early years of the pandemic, the condition was typically described as a 'gay plague', due to the fact that its first recorded recipients were men who had sex with men. This false impression, created by the initial pattern of the disease, had serious adverse implications for health promotion and the population at large. To many sections of society, homosexual men were perceived as a form of underclass whose illnesses were a 'just reward' for behaviour that was often not acceptable to the population in general. In many societies, sexual intercourse between consenting adult men was against the law, and/or contrary to the beliefs of a number of religions. As such, the views of the public at large – and politicians, in particular – were largely opposed to any public resources being directed towards health promotion activity to assist such a vulnerable section of the global community. When HIV/AIDS began to emerge within the drug misusing population, similar views were expressed regarding the development of health promotion measures targeted at this section of society. These views were challenged by a growing collation of health professionals, including nurses, and self-help groups – particularly in the USA and the UK. In the next section of this chapter, we will consider how two of the main health promotion strategies developed, and the ethical and political challenges they faced.

Additional point

The United Nations AIDS Organization website contains a detailed breakdown of the current prevalence of HIV/AIDS across the world. The website also contains information regarding the UN supported HIV prevention programmes.

The context of HIV/AIDS and drug misuse

Almost twenty years ago, in Liverpool in the UK, a group of public health practitioners challenged traditional views around HIV/AIDS; their actions led to the formation of the International Harm Reduction Association (IHRA). The IHRA has grown considerably since its early days and is now an organization that is acknowledged as a credible source of expertise by international agencies such as the WHO and governments around the globe. For example, the UK's Department for International Development provides funding to support the IHRA's networks. The IHRA supports harm reduction and health promotion programmes in every continent. It also has a network supporting service users. IHRA's latest network is the International Nursing Harm Reduction Network, whose members come from throughout the world.

Health promotion in action

The IHRA nursing network has hosted satellite seminars for nurses at the last three IHRA conferences in Vancouver, Warsaw and Barcelona. These seminars have enabled nurses to share the lessons they have gained through research and practice.

Led by Professor John Ashton (Regional Director of Public Health and Regional Medical Officer for the North West, UK) and Howard Seymour (Head of Health Promotion for Liverpool), a programme of innovative measures was introduced to limit the harm HIV might do to the local population. Their programme utilized a combination of primary and secondary prevention measures as the basis of the health promotion campaign. Primary measures were aimed at informing the general population about measures they could take to reduce their risk of exposure to HIV. However, it was their secondary prevention campaign that caused most controversy. At the heart of the health promotion campaign was the concept of harm reduction. Ashton and Seymour and their partners recognized that it was unrealistic to expect young adults to abstain from sexual intercourse, or drug users with addiction problems to stop using drugs. Therefore, their approach focused on reducing the riskiest forms of behaviour and, in consequence, reduce the chances of transmission of blood-borne viruses such as HIV (Ashton and Seymour 1993; Whitehead 2005).

The concept of harm reduction is based on the idea that the promotion of health is not an absolute but, rather, a continuum. The harm reduction approach recognizes that many people face circumstances that limit their ability to make major changes in their lives. However, by means of small, targeted steps, people can make incremental changes in their behaviour that will have positive benefits in their lives. These steps are aimed at reducing the most risky behaviour and providing a platform for future progress. The view of the IHRA is based on a balance between a pragmatic public health approach and a human rights approach. These views can be seen at www.ihra.net/whatisharmreduction However, some governments, law enforcement agencies, and religious groups across the world have challenged the approach of the IHRA and its supporters. Oliver (2006) summarized the international debate regarding decriminalization or prohibition of drugs such as heroin, cocaine and cannabis. Supporters of decriminalization argue it is because drug use is illegal that its victims get caught up in crimes such as theft, violence and prostitution. As the most commonly used illicit drug is cannabis – with ten times as many users compared with opiates – otherwise law abiding members of the public are classed as criminals. For people with addictions to illicit drugs, such as cocaine or heroin, the desire to seek help from health agencies is offset by the social and criminal justice consequences of their drug use becoming public knowledge. Oliver (2006) presents the arguments in favour of legalization, which include:

- The 'war on drugs' has been lost and society should not continue to waste resources in pursuit of failed prohibition policies
- Criminal law should not be used to inhibit personal freedom to use the drug of choice in private and personal circumstances that cause no harm to others
- The removal of profits from the drug trade would put suppliers and dealers out of business and thus end crime associated with suppliers and dealers
- Prohibition of alcohol in the USA did not work
- The actual harm in the form of deaths and related health problems is less than that caused by other 'legal' drugs – alcohol and tobacco

Studies to identify the hidden levels of substance misuse in a community, such as that of Beynon et al. (2001), demonstrate the challenge to effective health promotion with drug users if those most in need are deprived of access to help from nurses and other health professionals.

Opposition to decriminalization is led by the US government, which has limited the development of harm reduction programmes such as needle/syringe exchange schemes within its borders and in other parts of the world. In his presentation to the IHRA conference in Warsaw in 2007, Carl Phillips, a USA based advocate of harm reduction, highlighted the challenges faced by health promotion campaigns in the US (Phillips 2007). He stressed that this adverse influence extended to campaigns to introduce harm reduction programmes for tobacco use. Oliver (2006) also cited arguments for prohibition such as:

- Legalization would lead to increased use, addiction and associated medical costs
- Legalization would produce a huge administrative bureaucracy
- The economic arguments of savings in the criminal justice system and tax revenues offsetting are flawed
- Legalizing drugs will not alter adverse effects such as irrational and violent behaviour, and legal drugs would have the same effects as illegal drugs
- The compassionate approach to drugs is to do everything possible to reduce addiction, not to make it easier

This lack of international consensus, regarding an effective strategy to tackle HIV/ AIDS and drugs is reflected in a report by Kroll (2002), written for a WHO supported international task team on injecting drug use. This report provided an analysis of a range of programmes and projects implemented by the UN and other agencies. These initiatives had the aim of assisting countries across the globe to address the problems of HIV/AIDS and drug use, including measures related to health promotion, treatment and care, and health policy development. Kroll (2002) noted that:

> The UN system at country level has to respond to a multitude of different factors such as the extent of the epidemic amongst injecting drug users, the characteristics of drug users, national laws, legal provisions and policies towards drug use and HIV/AIDS, public opinions, involvement and interests of different public sectors, and the development and status of civil society organizations.

Injecting drug users provide a useful platform to expose the concept of harm reduction, and associated needle/syringe exchange programmes provide a good example of the political and ethical support for this form of health promotion. Analysis of injecting behaviour amongst drug users has highlighted that the sharing of injecting equipment was the main source of infection (Health Protection Agency 2003) As it is unlikely that injecting drug users would give up the use of drugs such as heroin because of their addiction to the drug, health promotion interventions focus on other aspects of their behaviour. In this case, the focus of health promotion interventions is on the sharing of injecting equipment. In the Liverpool initiative, syringe exchange schemes were established to enable drug users to gain access to free needles and syringes, thereby reducing the need to share such equipment. Health promotion programmes in this area generally promote the use of such exchanges, as well as messages about avoiding sharing injecting equipment. As part of a prescribed treatment programme, a second phase of the Liverpool initiative saw the introduction of methadone as a substitute for heroin. The idea behind this programme was to switch individuals from injecting heroin to the use of safer oral methadone. While it did not end the addiction to drugs, it did move the individual away from the high risk behaviour of injecting drug use to a relatively safer behaviour.

Tutorial brief 7.1

What are the possible ethical considerations behind a technique such as harm reduction, if it appears to condone an illegal behaviour?

Both these measures were seen as controversial at the time of their introduction but are now seen as mainstream measures in both the UK government's national drug strategy (National Treatment Agency for Substance Misuse 2004) and the Canadian governments Drug Strategy (Health Canada 2002). The techniques have been adopted across the globe and have contributed to a reduction in the spread of blood-borne viruses. Yet, in countries such as the United States, while the use of methadone substitution treatment has been adopted wholeheartedly, syringe exchange schemes have not been fully developed. (Drucker 1999; WHO 2004). Oliver (2006) reported on the intervention of the former US 'drugs czar' General McCaffrey, who blocked Federal funding of needle exchange programmes. General McCaffrey's rationale appeared to be based on his interpretation of Canadian data that indicated that old injecting equipment was not being exchanged for new material, and that injecting drug users were merely gaining free supplies. In Russia, substitution therapy using methadone is illegal, despite a rising number of drug users and a significant level of infections for HIV/AIDS. However, there is a growing number of needle/syringe exchange programmes, and there is limited use of another form of substitution therapy – in this case Buprenorphine (Alford et al. 2005) Health professionals, including nurses, are advocating policy changes to the Russian government to enable the less expensive but effective methadone programme to be legalized, as it will enable more drug users to access treatment and funds to be released for health promotion programmes to prevent the spread of blood-borne viruses. In some Eastern European countries, such as Lithuania, syringes and needles are widely available but drug users must pay for them (Kroll 2002). It can be seen here that a wide variance is presented concerning how to manage emotive high risk health promotion programmes between countries. This, in itself, presents its own dilemmas.

In Canada, the city of Vancouver opened the first 'supervised' injecting room for drug users in 2005. Supervised injecting rooms take the concept of harm reduction one stage further by enabling drug users to take their drugs in a clinic supervised by nurses. This approach means that, not only do drug users have access to sterile equipment, but they are also at reduced risk of overdose; overdose is a relatively common cause of death amongst drug users. The plan had been for similar sites to open in other parts of Canada, such as Toronto, as well as in North American cities such as Seattle. However, political opposition prevented the other centres from being established. A key difference in Vancouver was the leadership of the then Mayor Larry Campbell. Now a Canadian Senator, Campbell has a unique political background, having been the former Fire Chief, and then Police Chief of Vancouver before being elected Mayor. Working closely with health professionals, he came to realize that punitive measures against drug users were ineffective, alienating and wasteful. Subsequently, drug services in Vancouver and their associated health promotion services are amongst the best evaluated in the world (Wood et al. 2003, 2008). Vancouver's approach to harm reduction has been held up internationally as an excellent example of what can be achieved. Yet, following Larry Campbell's election to the Senate, a new political administration has come to power in the city. This administration seems less convinced of the merits of these harm reduction schemes (Maxwell 2007). Several factors underpin this different stance. One is economic, as these health promotion measures are not cheap. They required skilled staff (mostly nurses) working 365 days a year, with services opened from early morning to late at night. Another factor is the economic development of Vancouver, partly linked to its being the site for a future winter Olympics. Areas of the city where many of Vancouver's street drug users live, and where most of the specialist drug services are located, are seen as prime development land for business and luxury housing.

Here, in one of the great cities of the world, can be seen the beneficial and not-so-beneficial effects of political change for some of the most disadvantaged communities. Fortunately, at present, the weight of evidence that has been generated by the research projects evaluating their effectiveness has worked in their favour and made it difficult for politicians who oppose the programmes to stop them.

In the Vancouver example, the lines between ethical and political factors might be seen to blur. For example, nurses teaching safer injecting techniques to drug users and supervising the injecting of illegal drugs could be seen as condoning a crime and encouraging continued drug use. It could also be argued that the nurses are enabling their patients to harm themselves and, as such, they are contravening the ethical principle first laid down for nurses by Florence Nightingale: first, do the patient no harm. Nurses in Vancouver are lobbying city and state politicians to keep the safer injecting site open. Users of the service support their campaign. Their campaign utilizes robust peer reviewed research to argue the case for continuation of a health promotion programme recognized by the IHRA. These nurses are challenging the views of one group of elected politicians to advocate for a continuation of a policy developed with the support of the opposition group of politicians. In this case, ethics and politics are interlinked, and nurses are at the forefront of health promotion actioning.

Health promotion in action

Vancouver hosts several innovative health promotion programmes to promote the health of drug users, particularly those who are homeless. All involve nurses as key agents of health promotion. These include the street nurse programme. 'Insite' is the first supervised injection centre in North America, with 'She Way' a specialist project targeting women and including pregnant women (www.vch.ca); a similar 'Street Health' programme is led by nurses in Toronto. All these programmes offer a harm reduction based approach to health promotion and offer support to the most socially isolated sections of the Canadian populations. 'SMASH' is a nurse-led health promotion and substance misuse treatment service working in Sefton, near Liverpool, in the UK. The nurses include public health and mental health trained specialists who work with individuals and groups of young people at risk from alcohol and drug use. Group work has included enabling young people to develop their own health promotion materials, including DVDs to be shown in local schools and youth clubs. The team also provides sexual health promotion advice and services where appropriate.

 Tutorial brief 7.2

Consider the importance of generating a sound evidence base to support health promotion practice. How can this evidence base be used to influence the opinion of politicians and local communities?

HIV/AIDS: sexual health

The other major cause of transmission of HIV is sexual intercourse. As previously mentioned, in the early phase of the noted pandemic of AIDS it was considered by many people only to affect men who have sex with men. This short-sighted assessment adversely affected the development of an effective sexual health promotion strategy across the globe. In addition, religious, moral and political factors have also adversely affected the development of health promotion interventions around the world. Take condom promotion as an example of these constraints. A World Health Organization fact sheet regarding the effectiveness of male condoms stated:

> Condoms are the only contraceptive method proven to reduce the risk of all sexually transmitted infections, including HIV. (WHO 2000)

The fact sheet highlighted that a government campaign in Thailand promoting 100 per cent condom use amongst sex workers produced dramatic improvements. Usage increased from 14 per cent in 1990 to 94 per cent in 1994, with a significant reduction in sexually transmitted infections, including HIV amongst Thai soldiers. At complete odds with this is the continuing stance from the Catholic Church that condoms should not be used. For them, sexual abstinence is the only acceptable form of protection from sexually transmitted diseases. Especially in sub-Saharan Africa, where many people are devout Catholics, this presents a real problem that will not easily be resolved. The Catholic Church is under increasing pressure from many international health promotion agencies to change its stance.

Another WHO fact sheet regarding sexual health (WHO 2002) sets out working definitions that were developed from a WHO convened international technical consultation on sexual health in 2002. Intriguingly, the fact sheet states that these definitions **'do not represent an official WHO position, and should not be used or quoted as WHO definitions'** (the bold text is taken directly from the fact sheet).

Tutorial brief 7.3

Why should the WHO be reluctant to take an official position on sexual health, having convened an international group to develop these definitions?

Though not an official WHO definition, it is worth recording a number of the statements that have a bearing on sexual health promotion (WHO 2002):

> Addressing sexual health at the individual, family, community or health system level requires integrated interventions by trained health providers and a functioning referral system. It requires a legal, policy and regulatory environment where the sexual rights of all people are upheld.

Yet, across the world there are nation states, cultures and religions that are critical of aspects of human sexuality. This criticism applies particularly to men who have sex with men, sex workers, and those who have sexual intercourse outside of marriage. Such disapproval has limited the health promotion activities, either by action or inaction. In the case of inaction, governments or official bodies have chosen to ignore the need for health promotion initiatives amongst such sections of their populations. Such inaction might due to political factors, or a belief that other areas of health promotion merit prioritization, especially if resources are limited. In contrast, there might be a deliberate policy to marginalize the needs of such vulnerable sections of the community. In a speech to students of Columbia University, New York, in September 2007, the President of Iran, Mahoud Ahmadinejad, is quoted by the BBC as saying:

> In Iran we don't have homosexuals like in your country. (http://news.bbc.co.uk/ 1/hi/world/middle-east/7010962.stm)

In contrast to this, though, Iran has developed a very progressive drug treatment service that has received praise from the IHRA at its conferences in Vancouver 2006 and Warsaw 2007 (Azarakhsh 2007).

Sub-Saharan Africa has the highest prevalence of HIV/AIDS in the world. The WHO reported that, in the last 25 years, more than 25 million people have died of AIDS, of whom nearly two thirds of them are from sub-Saharan Africa. (WHO 2006) Of particular concern to WHO is the disproportionate impact on young women, with nearly three young women infected for every young man (15–24 year olds). The report also highlighted that, despite a UN General Assembly target of 90 per cent of people having knowledge about HIV by 2005, less than 50 per cent of young people are knowledgeable. However, in eight of the 11 African countries surveyed, the proportion of young people having sex before age 15 has declined and condom use has increased. While this appears to be good news, the prevalence of HIV in sub-Saharan Africa is such that a far greater improvement is needed, as Caroline Bradbury-Jones' analysis of the HIV/AIDS situation in Africa illustrates in Chapter 8.

The WHO (2006) HIV/AIDS report identifies a range of health promotion priorities including:

- Prevention of sexual transmission of HIV
- Prevention for people living with HIV/AIDS
- Prevention of HIV transmission through injecting drug use (harm reduction)

The report also identifies the importance of focusing efforts in areas where the organization has a sound evidence base for effective health promotion interventions.

In contrast to the WHO statements, the former president of the Republic of South Africa appears to have concerns about outside influences on his country. President Thabo Mbeki was also quoted by the BBC as stating, in 2000:

> It is obvious that whatever lessons we might have to draw from the West about the grave issue of HIV-AIDS, a simple superimposition of Western experience on

African reality would be absurd and illogical. I am convinced that our urgent task is to respond to the specific threat that faces us as Africans. We will not eschew this obligation in favour of the recitation of a catechism that might very well be a correct response to the specific manifestation of AIDS in the West. (http://news.bbc.co.uk)

In President Mbeki's letter to world leaders, he appeared to reject the advice from Western governments in relation to the how his country is dealing with the high levels of HIV/AIDS in his country on the basis that:

- HIV is a heterosexual not homosexual issue in South Africa
- Few people have died of AIDS in the West, while millions are said to have died in Africa
- AIDS deaths in the West are declining, whereas in Africa even greater numbers are destined to die.

Yet, sub-Saharan Africa has accepted high levels of HIV prevention funding through WHO and other Western agencies, including charitable funding from non-governmental organizations (NGOs). Such criticism from President Mbeki might also need to be viewed in the light of the funding shortage that has been highlighted in the Towards Universal Access by 2010 Report (WHO 2006). Here, the WHO identified that, in order to implement its plan, a budget of US$281 million would be needed in 2006–07: only US$161 million had been donated by member states and other donors.

Health promotion in action

In Burkina Faso, nurses have been an active part of a health promotion programme to reduce mother to child transmission (MTCT) of HIV/AIDS. Acknowledging the influential role religious leaders have within this community, a local nurse obtained permission from the Burkina Faso Assemblies of God national church to train over 100 of its pastors with regard to MTCT and the use of health promotion material that he had developed. The booklet was designed to contain a high number of drawings to enable users with low literacy skills. A follow-up study has shown the positive benefits from this approach to health promotion (Santmyire et al. 2006).

 Tutorial brief 7.4

What evidence is there to suggest that Western based organizations have tried to influence the public health policy of African states?

💭 **Tutorial brief 7.5**

To what extent should external agencies that fund health promotion programmes carried out by nurses be able to influence those programmes? Should the concept of 'he who pays the piper calls the tune' apply? What if the funding body is a commercial company: does that alter the situation?

Sex workers (often referred to as 'prostitutes' or 'hookers') are a group of women and men who sell sex for money. The reasons they do so are varied, although in many cases it is due to the need to fund a drug addiction. This need for money can pressurize sex workers to agree to undertake the riskier forms of sexual behaviour, as their clients will pay more for unprotected intercourse. Such behaviour places both sex workers and their clients at greater risk of sexually transmitted infections, including HIV. The views of European governments are mixed in relation to the best approach to address sexual health promotion amongst this group and their clients. Countries, such as Holland and Germany, have decriminalized or legalized prostitution, whereas Sweden has criminalized all aspects of street sex working (Home Office 2006). In the UK, the government conducted an extensive consultation exercise regarding its future strategy (Home Office 2006). Public and political opinions were mixed regarding whether legislation should be tightened or relaxed. Professional groups (such as the Royal College of Nursing) and advocacy groups (such as the English Collective of Prostitutes) argued the case for decriminalization. Both organizations were concerned that a tightening of the legislation would push sex working 'underground', making it more dificult for nurses and other health professionals to make contact with sex workers and their clients. Such legislation, they argued, would reduce the opportunity for sex workers to access health promotion advice or nurse led sexual health services for fear of prosecution. However, while the majority of the feedback the government received supported decriminalizing street sex working, it chose to develop a strategy that ignored this opinion (Home Office 2006).

In Liverpool, following the murder of two young female sex workers, local politicians agreed that something had to be done to reduce the risk to sex workers and the community at large. In a radical move, they agreed a cross-party approach to the issue and a major consultation exercise was undertaken within the city regarding the possible development of a managed zone for street sex working similar to those in Holland and New Zealand. A managed zone is a designated area where sex workers and their clients can meet without fear of prosecution. Health services including sexual health and blood-borne virus prevention are available and are often led by nurses. The consultation was carried out by Liverpool John Moores University and surveyed local residents, businesses, statutory agencies, voluntary sector organizations and, most importantly, sex workers themselves (Bellis et al. 2007) Their study demonstrated that there was a very high level of support across all the groups surveyed, and that the need for effective health promotion and better access to health services were seen as key reasons for this support. However, despite this research and the request from the city council to pilot a managed zone, the national government declined to permit this innovative public health measure to be trialled.

Health promotion in action

In Holland and New Zealand, the national governments and local councils have adopted a different approach to street prostitution compared with the UK and the USA. This has enabled sex workers to work in comparative safety. It has also enabled nurses and other health professionals to have easier access to carry out health promotion programmes related to sexual health and substance misuse. Jordan's (2005) review has reported the benefits in New Zealand of legislation that has enabled health workers to have better quality access to sex workers and their clients. Representatives from the Royal College of Nursing, the English Collective of Prostitutes and outreach workers from New Zealand and Sweden conducted a briefing to elected members of the UK's House of Commons and House of Lords to highlight the challenges faced in promoting the health of sex workers due to draft legislation going through the UK Parliament.

Additional information

The Scottish Parliament is also considering new legislation in relation to street prostitution. A new government in Holland is considering changing its more tolerant approach to street prostitution.

 ## Tutorial brief 7.6

What factors might have influenced the local and national governments to take differing positions on the issue of street sex working?

Summary point

Sexual health promotion is arguably one of the most challenging areas of health promotion due to the complex relationships with religion and culture, as well as the issues of sexual exploitation. Whereas the sexual exploitation of children has widespread condemnation, there are more diverse views in relation to what is perceived as the sexual exploitation of adults or acceptable behaviour between consenting adults. Prostitution can be said to typify this contrast and controversy. Child prostitution is a crime across the globe, but adult prostitution can be a criminal offence in one country and legitimate business in another. For nurses attempting to promote sexual health against a backdrop of rising sexually transmitted infections, the divergent views of different sectors of society and the different legislative frameworks present significant challenges for them and their patients.

Conclusion

Many areas of health promotion are not contentious and, therefore, have high levels of public and political support; for example, prevention of heart disease and strokes. However, there is a range of other topics that provoke controversy and leave nurses and other health promoters with ethical challenges. Using HIV/AIDS as an example of such topics, this chapter has outlined the local, national and international dimensions of these complex and challenging issues. These health challenges often have a disproportionate effect on the most vulnerable sections of societies, who often have the poorest access to health services and the weakest voice amongst the many voices calling for help or political change. The recent research carried out by Dahlgren and Whitehead, on behalf of the European office of the WHO, highlights this situation, even amongst the relatively affluent parts of Europe. (Dahlgren and Whitehead 2007; Whitehead and Dahlgren 2007) They describe the concept of a 'levelling up' approach to tackling health inequalities in order to ensure the health of the whole population is promoted and improved to the standard of the top 20 per cent. This concept, and those of human rights and harm reduction are at the heart of an ethical approach to health promotion. These concepts are also at the heart of any political advocacy that nurses might support in order to achieve change in the policies of governments, and for nurses to be given the resources they need to carry out effective public health programmes appropriate to the needs of the communities they serve. Each of these concepts recognizes that the balance of rights, needs, responsibilities and aspirations of individuals and communities. These concepts also acknowledge that health promotion and those nurses who undertake it play an important role in achieving the goals of the Ottawa Charter. As the Taiwanese Nurses Ethical Code of Conduct (2006) emphasizes:

> Nurses shall be concerned about the social, economic, environmental, and political factors that would affect health, and aggressively participate in advocating and promoting related policies according to their own specialities.

Health promotion is not merely a passive role for nurses delivering health information messages to our patients. It includes shaping the ethical and policy frameworks that influence the lives of our fellow citizens, and assertively advocating within the political structures of our countries for the legislative and financial resources to have a positive influence on the health and social well-being of our communities. This chapter also considers the ethical underpinning of nursing practice and the political factors that might affect the resources to support the health promotion programmes that they undertake. The chapter has considered examples from several countries across the world of the various HIV/AIDS related health promotion and disease prevention programmes. The chapter has reflected on the different approaches being taken by countries with similar cultural and political backgrounds – for example, Canada/UK/USA/New Zealand – as well as examples from Asia and Africa.

Summary point

This chapter has taken the subject of the HIV/AIDS pandemic to explore the issue the ethics and politics, and their impact on health promotion policy and practice for nurses and other health practitioners. The following key themes have been explored:

- Drug misuse
- Sexual health promotion
- Harm reduction
- Advocacy

Additional resources

American Nursing Association: http://nursing-world.com

Asia Regional HIV/AIDS Project 'HIV Awareness Raising and Community Based Effective Approaches', Burnet Institute Australia.

Association of Public Health Observatories (UK): www.apho.org.uk

Canadian Ministry of Health (2001) 'Best Practices for Treatment and Rehabilitation of Women with Substance Use Problems'.

Canadian Nursing Association: www.cna-nurses.ca

International Council of Nurses (ICN): www.icn.ch

Open Society Institute: Public Health Programme (2006) 'Fostering Enabling Legal and Policy environ-ments for Sex Workers' Health and Human Rights: A Compendium of Materials and Documents Addressing Sex Work, Health, Advocacy, Law and Human Rights.

Östergren, P. (2006) 'Sex Workers Critique of Swedish Prostitution Policy'. Available at www.petraoster-gren.com

Royal College of Nursing of Australia: www.rcna.org.au

Royal College of Nursing (UK): www.rcn.org.uk

Sidell, M., Jones, L., Katz, J., Peberdy, A. and Douglas, J. (2003) 'Debates and Dilemmas in Promoting Health: A Reader', 2nd edn (Basingstoke: Palgrave).

Terence Higgins Trust: www.tht.org.uk

Tilford, S., Delaney, F. and Vogels, M. (1997) 'Effectiveness of Mental Health Promotion Interventions: A Review' (London: Health Education Authority).

United Nations Millennium Goals: www.un.org/millenniumgoals

United Nations AIDS Organisation: www.unaids.org

British Medical Association (2008)
British Broadcasting Corporation (2007)
International Harm Reduction Association (n.d.)
Royal College of Nursing (n.d.)
Vancouver Coastal Health (n.d.)
United Nations (2001)
www.bma.org.uk/ap.nsf/Content/MedProfhumanRightsRecommendations
www.http://news.bbc.co.uk
www.ihra.net/whatisharmreduction
www.rcn.org.uk/learningzone – for information on specific political leadership programmes for nurses interested in being politically active.
www.vch.ca
www.un.org/millenium/declaration/ares552e.pdf – for the Millennium Development Goals (MDGs)

References

Alford, D.P., Labelle, C.T., Richardson, J.M. and O'Connell, J.J. et al. (2005) 'Treating Homeless Opioid Dependent Patients with Buprenorphine in an Office-based Setting', *Journal of General Internal Medicine*, 22(2): 171–6.

Antrobus, S. and Kitson, A. (1999) 'Nursing Leadership: Influencing and Shaping Health Policy and Nursing Practice', *Journal of Advanced Nursing*, 29: 745–53.

Ashton, J. and Seymour, H. (1993) *The New Public Health* (Buckingham: Open University Press).

Azarakhsh, M. (2007) 'Substitution Treatment in Iran', IHRA Conference, Warsaw.

Bellis, M.A., Watson, F.L.D., Hughes, S., Cook, P.A., Downing, J., Clark, P. and Thomson, R. (2007) 'Comparative Views of the Public, Sex Workers, Businesses and Residents on Establishing Managed Zones for Prostitution: Analysis of a Consultation in Liverpool', *Health and Place*, 13(3): 603–16.

Beynon, C., Bellis, M.A., Miller, T., Meier, P., Thomson, R. and Jones, K.M. (2001) 'Hidden Need for Drug Treatment Services: Measuring Levels of Problematic Drug Use in the North West of England', *Journal of Public Health Medicine*, 23(24): 286–91.

Chiou-Fen Lin, Meei-Shiow Lu, Hsien-Hsien Chiang, Chun-Chih Chung, Tze-Luen Lin, Teresa J.C. Yin and Che-Ming Yang (2007) 'Using a Citizen Consensus Conference to Revise the Code of Ethics for Nurses in Taiwan', *Journal of Nursing Scholarship*, 39(1): 95–101.

Clay, T. (1987) *Nurses: Power and Politics* (London: Heinemann Nursing).

Dahlgren, G. and Whitehead, M. (2007) European Strategies for Tackling Social Inequities in Health: Levelling Up Part 2', WHO Collaborating Centre (Europe), Liverpool University.

Drucker, E. (1999) 'Drug Prohibition and Public Health: 25 Years of Evidence', *Public Health Reports*, 114(1): 14–29 (Oxford: Oxford University Press).

Health Canada (2002) *Best Practices – Methadone Maintenance Treatment*, Canadian Ministry of Health.

Health Protection Agency (2003) 'Shooting Up: Infections among Injecting Drug Users in the UK'. Available online at www.hpa.gov.org.uk

Home Office (2006) 'A Co-ordinated Prostitution Strategy and a Summary of Responses to *Paying the Price*' (London: COI).

ICN (1998) *Nurses and Human Rights: Position Statement* (Geneva: ICN).

ICN (2000) 'Nursing Matters: ICN on Mobilising Nurses for Health Promotion' (Geneva: ICN). Available online at www.icn.ch/pshumanrights.htm

IHRA (2007) 'What is Harm Reduction?'. Available online at www.ihra.net

Jordan, J. (2005) *The Sex Industry in New Zealand: A Literature Review* (New Zealand: Ministry of Justice).

Kroll, C. (2002) 'Assistance to Country Responses on HIV/AIDS to Injecting Drug Use by the UN and Other Agencies', Report for the Inter Agency Task Team on Injecting Drug Use (Vienna: World Health Organization).

Maxwell, G. (2007) 'The Threat to INSITE, Vancouver's Supervised Injection Site', Abstract 707, IHRA Conference, Warsaw.

National Treatment Agency for Substance Misuse (2004) 'Service Specification Tier 3: Community Prescribing' (London: NTA, Royal College of General Practitioners).

NMC (2008) 'The Code: Standards, Conduct, Performance and Ethics for Nursing and Midwives' (London: Nursing and Midwifery Council).

Oliver, I. (2006) *Drug Affliction: What You Need To Know* (Aberdeen: Robert Gordon University Press).

Oxford English Dictionary of Current English (2002) 2nd edn (Oxford: Oxford University Press).

Phillips, C. (2007) 18th International Conference on the Reduction of Drug-Related Harm. Available at http://www.aids.md/files/events/2007/808/conference-programme-overview.pdf

Rothstein, W. and Phuong, L. (2007) 'Ethical Attitudes of Nurse, Physician and Unaffiliated Members of Institutional Review Boards', *Journal of Nursing Scholarship*, 39(1): 75–81.

Santmyire, A. and Jamison, M. (2006) 'Educating African Pastors on Mother-to-Child Transmission of HIV/AIDS', *Journal of Nursing Scholarship*, 38(4): 321–7.

Scriven, A. and Orme, J. (eds) (2001) *Health Promotion: Professional Perspectives*, 2nd edn (Basingstoke: Palgrave).

Snow, T. (2009) 'This Year's Challenge: Maintaining Quality Care under a Tight Budget', *Nursing Standard*, 7 January, 23(18).

Whitehead, D. (2003) 'The Health-Promoting Nurse as a Health Policy Career Expert and Entrepreneur', *Nurse Education Today*, 23: 585–92.

Whitehead, D. (2005) 'In Pursuit of Pleasure: Health Education as a Means of Facilitating the "Health Journey" of Young People', *Health Education*, 105: 213–27.

Whitehead, M. and Dahlgren, G. (2007) 'Concepts and Principles for Tackling Social Inequities in Health: Levelling Up Part 1', WHO Collaborating Centre (Europe), Liverpool University.

WHO (2000) 'Effectiveness of Male Latex Condoms in Protecting against Pregnancy and Sexually Transmitted Infections' (Geneva: WHO).

WHO (2002) 'Sexual Health'. Available online at www.who.int/reproductive-health/gender/sexualhealth.html

WHO (2004) 'Outcome Evaluation Summary Report: WHO/UNODC Global Initiative (1999–2003) on Primary Prevention of Substance Abuse' (Geneva: WHO).

WHO (2006) *Towards Universal Access by 2010* (Geneva: WHO).

Wood, E., Spittal, P.M., Kerr, T., Small, W., Tyndall, M.W., O'Shaughnessy, M.V. and Schechter, M.T. (2003) 'Requiring Help Injecting is a Risk Factor for HIV Infection in the Vancouver Epidemic: Implications for HIV Prevention', *Canadian Journal of Public Health*, September–October, 94(5): 355–559.

Wood, E., Stoltz, J.A., Zhang, R., Strathdee, S.A., Montaner, J.S., Kerr, T. (2008) 'Circumstances of First Crystal Methamphetamine Use and Initiation of Injecting Drug Use amongst High-Risk Youth', *Drug Alcohol Review*, May, 27(3): 270–6.

CHAPTER 8

Current and Future Developments in Health Promotion

Caroline Bradbury-Jones

Objectives

By the end of this chapter you should be able to:

- Identify the most significant health issues in contemporary society
- Understand the implications of globalization on health
- Debate the benefits and challenges to health that arise as a result of globalization
- Understand the importance of viewing health through a global lens
- Identify the global policy framework that underpins contemporary health promotion practice
- Explore improvements to global health achieved during recent decades and opportunities for future progress
- Understand how current and future developments in health promotion might impact on nursing

---

Key terms

- Globalization
- Health policy
- Inequalities in health
- Inter-sectoral collaboration
- Millennium Declaration
- Millennium Development Goals

Introduction

Over the last century, life expectancy has increased considerably across the world, and there has been a corresponding decline in child deaths. This contemporary profile of global mortality represents a decline in death rates that began in the eighteenth century.

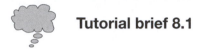 **Tutorial brief 8.1**

Think about the decline in death rates over the past few centuries. Before reading on, what do you think are the primary reasons for the reduction? Make a list of your ideas.

McKeown (1979) undertook an analysis of the reasons for the increase in population in England and Wales during the eighteenth century, which for many years had been attributed to a decline in mortality brought about by medical advances alone. He challenged this viewpoint by asserting that, with the exception of smallpox, medical interventions such as immunization and treatment had contributed little to the reduction of deaths from infectious diseases. Instead, he considered that health was transformed during the eighteenth century because of improved nutrition, better hygiene and contraception. Therefore, for the past few decades, it has become established wisdom that improvements in the health profile of Western populations since the 1800s have resulted primarily from broad-based changes in the social, dietary and material environment – shaped, at least in part, by improved sanitation and other deliberate public health interventions (McMichael and Beaglehole 2003). There has subsequently been a corresponding change to the face of public health. According to Peersman (2001), public health has now gained a broader vision that deals with major health issues such as the environment, sanitation and living conditions. The reason for this is quite simple: if better health is achieved as a result of sanitation rather than immunization, there must be a broad view of the determinants and, indeed, the sustainability of population health (McMichael and Beaglehole 2003).

Summary point

Over the past few centuries, life expectancy has increased and this is mostly attributable to overall improvements in the environment, sanitation and living conditions.

It might appear contradictory to begin a chapter that is concerned with current and future developments in health promotion with a historical perspective. However, the aim of this chapter is to focus on the changing health profile of the global population, as the most challenging – and, arguably, visible – current and future agenda for health promotion. One way of understanding the present and future situation of health promotion is to situate it initially within its historical context. There are three issues that form the core discussion in this chapter: globalization, inequalities in health, and shifting patterns of health. It is only through an understanding of these complex and interrelated issues that effective contemporary and future health promotion programmes can be developed. The chapter concentrates on global issues relating to health and, by necessity, has a broad focus. Implications for nursing are discussed but, congruent with the rest of the chapter, these are also explored within the broad context of nursing as a whole, rather than focusing on individual nurses' practice.

Improvements in global health

There is an unsurprising relationship between the increasing life expectancy referred to in the opening section of this chapter and overall improvements in global health. For example, at the beginning of the twentieth century smallpox was still endemic in almost every country in the world but, through the efforts of a worldwide campaign, the World Health Organization certified the global eradication of smallpox in 1979 (WHO 2007a). More recently, at a global level reported on by the United Nations (UN 2007), the tuberculosis epidemic finally appears to be on the verge of decline. In relation to measles, deaths fell by over 60 per cent between 2000 and 2005, the most striking gains being in Africa, where measles deaths decreased by nearly 75 per cent over the same period. According to Mathers and Loncar (2006), the positive trends in reduction of such communicable diseases are set to continue and large declines in mortality are projected for TB, malaria and other infectious diseases between 2002 and 2030. Although such achievements make for heartening reading, the profile of worldwide health continues to alter with varying proportions of winners and losers. As some diseases are eliminated, new ones emerge in their place – for example, HIV and AIDS: these still constitute a significant challenge to the health of people world-wide. Ironically, increases in life expectancy can represent a double-edged sword, in that longevity brings with it individual and social challenges of its own. It is to these very issues that this chapter now turns its attention.

Shifting patterns of health

 Tutorial brief 8.2

As the title of this section indicates, the past century has seen some significant changes in the health of the world's population. Draw a line down the middle of a blank piece of paper to form two columns. In one column make a list of the ways in which the health of the population has improved during this time and, in the other, make a list of the ways it has declined. Try to write down at least several items in each column.

Projected figures are that the ageing of the global population will result in significant increases in the total number of deaths caused by non-communicable diseases
in the next thirty years (WHO 2007b). The same figures predict large declines in
mortality expected to occur for all of the principal communicable causes between
2002 and 2030, with the exception of HIV/AIDS. Overall, though, the pattern is
such that non-communicable conditions will account for almost 70 per cent of all
deaths in 2030. Of these, ischaemic heart disease, cerebro-vascular disease and
chronic obstructive pulmonary disease will be the leading causes of death, along
with HIV/AIDS. In essence, the global pattern for the next few decades is that
communicable diseases, as the current most serious health threat, will be overtaken
by non-communicable diseases, with the latter posing a significant challenge to the
health of people worldwide. This changing pattern is largely attributable to lifestyle
factors, a fuller discussion of which was provided in Chapter 1.

Summary point

With the exception of HIV/AIDS, communicable diseases are no longer
the most serious threat to health for the world's population. Instead, non-
communicable diseases account for most morbidity and mortality, particularly ischaemic heart disease, cerebro-vascular disease and chronic
obstructive pulmonary disease.

HIV/AIDS is a known anomaly in the shift from communicable to non-communicable diseases as being the most important health threat for people today. In a
short space of time, HIV/AIDS has grown from being something (incorrectly)
associated as affecting only minority communities – such as injecting drug users, sex
workers and gay men – to become the most serious pandemic the world has ever
known (Aggleton 2005). From the global health trends noted so far in this chapter,
it appears that measures to prevent the spread of HIV are having little effect. In fact,
the number of people with HIV/AIDS is likely to increase by nearly four million
over the next twenty years (UN 2007; WHO 2007b). Inequalities in health will be
explored later in the chapter, but they are never more evident than in relation to the
distribution and spread of HIV/AIDS. There exists an uneven distribution of the
disease globally with sub-Saharan Africa continuing to bear the brunt of the global
epidemic. Two thirds of all adults and children with HIV live in sub-Saharan Africa,
with an estimated one-in-three adults living with HIV in 2005 in Swaziland alone
(UNAIDS/WHO 2006). It is a stark reality that, despite global increases in average
life expectancy, some sub-Saharan countries now have inferior life expectancy rates
than they did a decade ago – mainly attributed to the scourge of HIV/AIDS
(McDaid and Oliver 2005). As one might expect, Chapter 7 too draws quite heavily
on HIV/AIDS related issues in order to illustrate a number of political and health
policy constructs.

    The discussion so far has pointed to the changing health profile of the worldwide
population, but this should not be viewed in isolation from other factors with which

it is inextricably linked. The WHO (2005) has acknowledged that many of the critical factors that now influence health include increasing inequalities within and between countries, and globalization. It is these two significant issues, coupled with a more in-depth exploration of the changing profile of global health, that need to be discussed in greater detail. These issues are discussed individually for the sake of clarity, but separating them in this way risks reductionism. In other words, there is a chance that the reader might perceive these issues to be readily separable entities: this is not the case. The issues have been reduced to individual parts solely to aid explanation but, as will be made clear as the chapter unfolds, globalization, inequalities and changing patterns of global health are very closely interrelated. They form a complex nexus that present a serious challenge, not only for individual health, but also for the nursing profession as a whole. While many nurses are still coming to terms with the last 'new' health promotion reforms that sought to promote more national and localized community development and community empowerment, in an attempt to shift 'health promotion' away from more traditional behavioural individual health education activities, there is now a need to realize that current and future reforms ask nurses to draw their attention also to activity at the global level.

Globalization

According to Scriven (2005), globalization describes the phenomenon of increased economic and social interdependence between countries. Jenkins (2004: 1) describes it as:

> a process of greater integration within the world economy through movements of goods and services, capital, technology and (to a lesser extent) labour, which lead increasingly to economic decisions being influenced by global conditions.

The interdependence produced by globalization has broken down traditional ways of conceptualizing and organizing the medical, economic, political and technological means to improve health (Drager and Fidler 2007). For example, in health promotion the globalization agenda emphasizes a shift from localized community activities (such as community development) to a much broader global collaborative approach. This indicates to nurses that they also need recognize this change of emphasis, which takes the reader now even further beyond the context of health promotion as discussed in Chapter 1.

 Tutorial brief 8.3

Globalization can impact on health both positively and negatively. Before reading any further, write two short statements: one on the way that you think globalization can positively affect health, and another about its potential negative influence on health.

To McMichael and Beaglehole (2003), economic globalization is a mixed blessing. For them, on one hand economic growth and technological advancement have improved life expectancy but, on the other hand, globalization is increasing the rich–poor gap and widening consumerism. In terms of the positive influences of globalization, one view is that it can create opportunities for cooperation to improve health and reduce global risks. Such opportunities include, for example, enhanced information and communications technology, and improved mechanisms for global governance and sharing of experiences (WHO 2005). Conversely, infectious diseases are spreading much faster geographically than at any time in history – and appear to be emerging more quickly than ever before. According to the WHO (2007a), there are now nearly forty diseases that were unknown a generation ago. The primary reason for the faster spread of diseases is the increasing mobility of the world's population, aided by advances in the global transport infrastructure. Severe acute respiratory syndrome (SARS) and avian influenza in humans have triggered major international concern, raised new scientific challenges, caused major human suffering and imposed enormous economic damage (WHO 2007a). There is a chance that avian and human influenzas could combine to create a pandemic influenza with the capability of spreading from human-to-human on a global scale (Alcock and Delieu 2007) – thus highlighting the challenges to health of globalization.

 Tutorial brief 8.4

Look at the two statements that you provided for Tutorial 8.3. On the basis of what you have written, what do you think are the implications for nursing?

Overall, governments agreed in the *Millennium Declaration* report that globalization should become a positive force for all (UN 2007). However, as noted by the UN General Assembly (2000), while globalization offers great opportunities, its benefits are unevenly shared and its costs unevenly distributed. In response to this, nurses need to be mindful of new health challenges to the global population and how they impact at the more local practice.

Inequalities in health

Health inequalities refer to differences in health status or in the distribution of health determinants between different populations (WHO 2007b). While overall health status worldwide, measured in terms of life expectancy, has continued to improve over the last fifty years, not all countries have benefited. As the new millennium began, the gap in health status between the poorest nations and those in wealthier countries was becoming wider (Davey 2005). For example, average life expectancy at birth ranges from 81.9 years in Japan to just 34 years in Sierra Leone

(McDaid and Oliver 2005): another stark illustration of global inequality. In addition to the global health inequality situation, while infant and child mortality rates have declined globally, the pace of progress remains uneven across countries. The vulnerability of children has increased and, additionally, over half a million women still die each year from treatable and preventable complications of pregnancy and childbirth – almost all of them in sub-Saharan Africa and Asia (WHO 2005; UN 2007).

Summary point

Health inequalities are the difference in health status experienced by different populations and countries. Despite the overall increases in life expectancy globally, health inequalities between countries persist. In fact, over the last few decades the gap between the richest and poorest countries has increased.

In terms of environmental factors influencing health, half the population of the developing world lack basic sanitation, and the provision of water for drinking and hygiene remains a huge challenge (UN 2007; WHO 2007a). The health, economic and social repercussions of open defecation, poor hygiene and lack of safe drinking water are well documented (UN 2007). Children bear the brunt of the effect of poor sanitation, and data from the WHO (2007a) suggest that more than 4500 children under five years of age die every day from easily preventable diseases such as diarrhoea. Moreover, infestation of intestinal worms caused by open defecation negatively affects children's physical fitness and cognitive function, which, in turn, have implications for school attendance, anaemia, and, for girls, increased risk of complications in childbirth (UN 2007).

Health promotion in action

Hosseinpoor et al. (2006) undertook a study that measured socioeconomic inequality in child/infant mortality in Iran. They found that a mother's illiteracy, risky birth interval and living in a rural area are more prevalent among low socioeconomic groups, and are associated with increased infant mortality risk. Conversely, they reported that having a hygienic toilet is associated with reduced risk of infant mortality. They concluded that health promotion action – in the form of investments in water, sanitation, and housing – could directly influence the reduction of inequality of child mortality, particularly in rural areas.

The link between inequalities and non-communicable diseases is complex. Non-communicable diseases remain a significant issue in affluent countries, but they are increasing most rapidly in developing countries. This means that the health profiles of developing and developed countries are beginning to look the same.

This transition is driven by the gradual reduction in childhood mortality from some major infectious diseases, as discussed earlier in the chapter, together with improved survival into adulthood that enables the ageing of the population (Davey 2005). The *relative* ageing of any population brings with it risks of non-communicable diseases such as coronary heart disease and diabetes, which is the case for all parts of the world. However, as will be explored later, globalization plays more than a small part in exacerbating the burden of disease associated with non-communicable diseases, particularly for the poorer regions of the world.

New patterns of health

There is a complex relationship between globalization and increases in non-communicable diseases. Importantly, the consumption of tobacco and alcohol is rising rapidly in developing countries (Davey 2005), a phenomenon that is largely associated with globalization. Beyond doubt, tobacco use is linked to serious health risks and mortality. At a worldwide level, tobacco consumption kills five million people per year and the rates are rising (Yach et al. 2005). However, morbidity and mortality associated with smoking are not distributed equally across the globe. Comparatively, it is the developing countries that carry the greatest burden of disease. The combination of higher prevalence of tobacco use and more limited access to health resources compound health inequalities (WHO 2007b).

In relation to health risks linked to nutrition, across the globe diets are becoming proportionately higher in fats and sugars and lower in dietary fibre (Yach et al. 2005). Perhaps, unsurprisingly, the result of this is that obesity has become a global issue. The health profile of developing countries in relation to nutrition is paradoxical however, because, on one hand, there is greater access to foods, (which, because of their composition, pose a health risk) yet, on the other hand, malnutrition due to insufficient and unsustained food supplies remains a serious health problem for many people. Perhaps unsurprisingly, children bear the highest risk of malnutrition and wasting. Wasting is a sign of acute malnutrition and is a strong predictor of mortality among children. According to the WHO (2007b), the global estimate of wasting in children under the age of five years is 10 per cent. The highest numbers of affected children live in south-central Asia, and many of them are likely to die before reaching the age of five years.

Summary point

Tobacco use and poor nutrition are implicated in relation to changing patterns of health across the globe. The situation in relation to nutrition is particularly complex in developing countries, where increasing rates of obesity run side-by-side with enduring problems of undernutrition – particularly in children.

Health promotion in action

The WHO (2003) has set out a number of measures aimed at reducing the risk of developing cardiovascular disease. The measures are based on available evidence and aim to promote health by: reducing dietary intake of fats, sodium and alcohol; enhancing dietary intake of fruit and vegetables, potassium, fibre and fish; and encouraging physical exercise. Full details of the recommendations are available on pages 87–91 of the report and are available online.

As discussed, so far, health in contemporary society is a complex issue and seemingly contradictory. We know that life expectancy is increasing, but that this is not equal across the globe. The world population is ageing, but this adds to the burden of disease associated with longevity. Globalization means that some developing countries have greater access to food supplies, but changing diets in these countries are associated with increasing rates of non-communicable diseases. Despite enhanced food security in some developing countries, many children still die from starvation. Such complexities pose a significant challenge to those interested in or wanting to practice health promotion. In identifying the issues underpinning global health as a major agenda for health promotion and health practitioners, this chapter can now explore the health-promoting strategies by which some of these challenges can be overcome in order to secure better health for the world's population.

Additional point

Some nurses might be inclined to think that the major global health issues mainly affect those working in developing nations. This, however, is a flawed perception, as it is clear to see that global health issues affect us all –how we practise and how our practices are resourced. Other influential global factors, such as the world economy and environmental concerns, help to illustrate this further.

Addressing challenges to global health

Inter-sectoral collaboration

There is clear consensus that, in order to address global health challenges, intersectoral collaboration is essential (Tones and Tilford 2001; Mittelmark 2005). In other words, there is a need for all health professionals, agencies and sectors to work together – with nursing needing to be as visible as possible.

Tutorial brief 8.5

Think about the health challenges already discussed in this chapter. With these in mind, write down: (1) the part that nursing can play in addressing these issues; (2) the issues that nursing cannot tackle alone.

The principal reason why inter-sectoral collaboration is important relates to the viewpoint of McKeown (1976). As discussed earlier, this is the view that health is determined by social, demographic and economic factors, and public policies that extend well beyond the traditional remit of medicine (Levin and Ziglio 2003). The consequence is that health promotion needs to go beyond traditional health services and put health on the agenda of policy-makers in all sectors, including public, private, non-governmental and international organizations (WHO 1986, 2005). Promoting health and, specifically, alleviating health inequalities cannot be achieved by the health sector in isolation. Instead, a broader approach is needed (McDaid and Oliver 2005). Moreover, according to Tones and Tilford (2001) there are significant gains in working together, not least because of the synergistic effect from 'joined-up' working. However, the challenges are that health promotion tends to be too insular (Mittelmark 2005). Additionally, health and environmental issues are inclined to occupy different worlds. Baggott (2000) suggests that this is reflected in the separation of responsibility for these issues between agencies at local, national and international level on matters that ought to be of mutual concern.

Health promotion in action

Bradsher et al. (2006) show how collaboration between international public health agencies and the Kenyan government had positive effects on the outcome of a vaccination programme. They report on the evaluation of a mass immunization campaign (the Measles Initiative) in Kenya that resulted in a reduction in measles incidence by more than 99 per cent. They attribute the success of the campaign directly to the collaboration of expert partners and agencies across the health care sector.

There are some important issues when considering inter-sectoral collaboration that are worthy of consideration. Firstly, the manner in which the health needs of communities and populations are assessed (see Chapter 4). Horne (2003) states that health needs assessment is about identifying need as perceived by people themselves, and developing solutions to the problems identified. She provides the example of Rapid Participatory Appraisal as one such approach. This involves engagement with key informants from the community in order to gain insight into the priority needs of the community from the community's perspective. What is important from this perspective is that a bottom-up approach is adopted in relation to health needs assessment.

A second issue for effective inter-sectoral collaboration relates to the evaluation of strategies, policies and programmes aimed at promoting health (see Chapter 4). These need to be assessed in terms of their impact on health. According to the UK Department of Health (DoH 2004), all such policies and programmes should be systematically appraised in the form of health impact assessment (HIA). This appraisal involves identifying and weighing up the costs and benefits of the policy or programme in relation to the impact on the population's health. Reflecting on earlier discussion in the chapter, and specifically on Tutorial brief 8.5, it will hope-fully be evident that the critical element in HIA is to consider all sectors, not merely nursing and health.

Summary point

Inter-sectoral collaboration is important because health is determined by social, demographic and economic factors. Therefore, effective health promotion relies on the 'joined-up' working of different agencies and organ-izations. The Ottawa and Bangkok charters are examples of policy at global level that aims to involve different agencies in promoting health.

Using international policy as the basis for health promotion

According to Drager and Fidler (2007), governments are charged with finding ways to manage health risks associated with globalization. They suggest that this creates the new world of 'global health diplomacy'. This is a term that refers to the relation-ship between health and foreign policy and, specifically, how countries need to orient such policies in ways that align national interests with globalized ones. Put simply, this means that countries need to consider other countries, and the actual and potential effects they have on each other. More often than not, this usually means the effects that developed and developing countries have on undeveloped countries, such as with 'global warming' and climate change.

From the early 1970s, the WHO has been a key organizational body for deter-mining the frameworks that dictate the nature and function of health promotion practice. As a response to the Alma–Ata Declaration on Health for All (WHO 1978), the Ottawa Charter for Health Promotion provided an initial framework for agreeing the activities needed to constitute health promotion practice (WHO, 1986). The Ottawa Charter was mainly a response to growing expectations for a global 'new public health movement'. It recognized the basic prerequisites for health as: peace, shelter, education, food, income, a stable eco-system, sustainable resources, social justice and equity. It also directed health promotion activity towards building healthy public policy, creating supportive environments, strengthening community action, developing personal skills, reorienting health services, and moving health promotion into the future.

The original Ottawa Charter has now been updated and built upon by the Bangkok Charter for Health Promotion in a Globalized World (WHO 2005). The Bangkok Charter complements and builds upon the principles and strategies established by the Ottawa Charter, but it acknowledges that the global context for health promotion has changed markedly since the development of the Ottawa Charter. The main change since the original charter is the move from localized community development towards globalization of health through *national capacity* (Catford 2005). National capacity means managing globalization through policy development and partnership building; provision of evidence-based examples of successful health promotion programmes; and global monitoring, reporting and capacity building initiatives for enhancing health promotion (Catford 2005). Nursing is being charged, alongside all health care agencies, with the responsibility of working towards this form of global reform of health care practice (Whitehead 2009). This chapter can now begin to explore the extent to which the various WHO charters, along with other policies, have had an influence on global health – with particular reference to changing patterns of health and inequalities in health.

Using policy to tackle changing patterns of health

According to Magnusson (2007), non-communicable diseases are a serious threat to health in both developed and developing countries, and deserve to be treated as a global health priority. The Ottawa Charter made a commitment to counteract the effects of unhealthy living conditions, environments and poor nutrition. Its core message was to make the healthier choice the easier choice – not solely for the population, but for policy-makers as well (WHO 1986). In terms of tackling the worldwide increase in non-communicable diseases attributable to smoking, this is important. For example, according to the WHO (2007c) there is clear evidence that the provision of smoke-free environments is the only effective way to reduce the harmful effects of exposure to second-hand tobacco smoke. But, in terms of ease of for policy-makers, smoke free environments only become the 'easy choice' when supported by legislation. It is legal – rather than voluntary – policies that are necessary. Passing legislation is not enough on its own; proper implementation and adequate enforcement are also necessary (WHO 2007c).

Health promotion in action

Sargent et al. (2004) report on a study undertaken in North America to determine whether enactment of legislation to require smoke-free workplaces and public places was associated with a decline in hospital admissions for acute myocardial infarction. They studied one community that had a ban for a limited period (six months). They found that, during this period, there was a significant reduction in admissions for myocardial infarction. They concluded that laws to enforce smoke-free environments might be associated with an effect on morbidity from heart disease.

In terms of changing global dietary patterns and the effect on health, policy at a global level is important, too. For example, obesity is not just an individual problem; it is a population problem. Tackling obesity requires an integrated approach involving all sectors of society; this is the inter-sectoral collaboration discussed earlier. Countries with developing economies require specific health promotion strategies because of the issues, already discussed, regarding co-existence of obesity and under-nutrition.

Using policy to tackle inequalities in health

International initiatives, directly or indirectly, can help to tackle inequalities in health; one such example is the Millennium Development Goals (MDGs). The MDGs were produced by the Organisation for Economic Cooperation and Development as a framework to guide policies and programmes across the globe. They are a universal framework for developing countries, and their partners to work together to secure a shared future for all (UN 2007). At their heart, they have a commitment to create an environment that is conducive to development and the reduction of poverty (Scriven 2005).

 ### Tutorial brief 8.6

Access the Millennium Development Goals online (available at http://devdata. worldbank.org/atlas-mdg/). Familiarize yourself with each of the targets. You might want to print off a copy for your file, or make a written note of each of the targets.

   The MDGs have a focus on health-promoting activities for low income countries – including, for example, objectives to eradicate extreme poverty and hunger; reducing child mortality; improving maternal health; and combating HIV/AIDS, malaria and other diseases (McDaid and Oliver 2005). One target of the MDGs is to halve the population of people without sustainable access to safe drinking water and sanitation by 2015 (WHO 2006). This is critical, given that, as discussed earlier, 1.1 billion people lack access to safe water and 2.6 billion people lack access to proper sanitation (WHO 2007a). One way of addressing this is through investments in water, sanitation and housing, which could directly reduce child mortality. This clearly illustrates how public health strategies that consider environmental health interventions are important, at both national and international levels. It also reinforces the point, made earlier, that health policies alone are insufficient for promoting health – particularly in reducing inequalities in health.

The (in)effectiveness of policies to promote health

According to the Bangkok Charter, government and international bodies must act to close the health gap between the rich and the poor (WHO 2005). In terms of poverty, there are indicators of success. For example, the proportion of people living in extreme poverty fell from nearly one third to fewer than one fifth between 1990 and 2004 and, in most developing regions, the average income of those living on less than $1 a day has increased (UN 2007). If this trend continues, the MDG poverty reduction target will be met for the world as a whole and for most regions. However, we are rapidly approaching the 2015 target date and the UN (2007) acknowledges that, although there has been some progress, there is still much to be done. According to Magnusson (2007), although financial and human resource constraints have created some setbacks, effective interventions need to be better targeted to the poor. Whether the MDGs can be attained and, furthermore, whether they will reduce inequalities in health has been questioned by McDaid and Oliver (2005). Their conclusion is that the current situation is discouraging. Half the developing world is without basic sanitation, and the target is to halve the proportion of people without sustainable access to safe drinking water and basic sanitation (UN General Assembly 2000). However, if trends continue, the target is likely to be missed (UN 2007).

Additionally, if current trends continue, the target of halving the proportion of underweight children will be missed, largely because of the slow progress in Southern Asia and sub-Saharan Africa (UN 2007). Indeed, in the case of the latter, at the current rate of progress it will take approximately 150 years to reach targets for the reduction of childhood mortality and poverty (McDaid and Oliver 2005). Overall, although there is evidence of success of contemporary policy in relation to reducing poverty and improving access to clean drinking water, there is still a great deal to be done. Unless political leaders take urgent action, many millions of people will not realize the basic promises of the MDGs in their lives (UN 2007). However, it is not only up to political leaders to realize global health. Nursing will be called upon to be a prominent force in the global community. Nurses will need to be at the forefront of the emerging global health promotion 'revolution'. This means concerted action at the international and national levels, and also at the local level. Even with the richer nations of the world comes the realization that there are national, regional and local levels of health inequity, poverty and high child mortality. Overarching all of this is the commonly used adage employed in an international context: 'without the health of my 'brother' [neighbour] there can be no health for me'.

Summary point

Although there appears to have been a rhetorical commitment at policy level to reduce inequalities in health, and to improve the determinants of health in developing countries, this does not appear to be reflected in practice. With only a few exceptions, even the commitment to achieving the MDGs within the projected timeframe seems unlikely.

Conclusion

Current and future developments in health promotion are dependent on an acknowledgement of the impact of globalization on health, recognition of the changing profile of global health and reducing inequalities in health. Additionally, there needs to be understanding that improving global health is a significant challenge and cannot be achieved by single actions or single agencies; neither can it be achieved through short-term measures alone. What this means for health promotion strategies is: first, a commitment by individual nurses and other health agencies to work collaboratively in order to tackle the broad determinants of health; second, a need to exercise patience.

A problem with initiatives to tackle inequalities in health is the time lag between implementing policies and their impact. Long-term planning is required to overcome 'political short-termism' (McDaid and Oliver 2005: 45), which risks giving up on potentially useful policies and strategies before they have had a chance to take effect. In terms of contemporary policies, we are fortunate to have in place the Ottawa and Bangkok Charters and the MDGs: potentially, these can act as drivers towards improving global health. Therefore, every opportunity needs to be seized and, as this book argues, particularly by nurses and nursing as a whole.

Additional resources

For more information on public health and the development of health promotion, see Naidoo, J. and Wills, J. (2000) *Health Promotion: Foundations for Practice*, 2nd edn (Edinburgh: Baillière Tindall and the Royal College of Nursing) ch. 9: 181–97.

Globalization is discussed in greater depth from an economic perspective in Mason, T. and Whitehead, E. (2003) *Thinking Nursing* (Maidenhead: Open University Press) ch. 7: 252–83.

References

Aggleton, P. (2005) 'HIV/AIDS: Lessons for and from Health Promotion' in Scriven, A. and Garman, S. (eds), *Promoting Health: Global Perspectives* (Basingstoke: Palgrave Macmillan): 115–28.

Alcock, J. and Delieu, J. (2007) 'Planning for Pandemic Influenza', *Nursing Standard*, 22(3): 35–9.

Baggott, R. (2000) *Public Health: Policy and Politics* (Basingstoke: Macmillan).

Bradsher, C.A., Stotts, R.C., Carter, M.A. and Grabowsky, M. (2006) 'The Measles Initiative to Control Measles in Kenya', *Public Health Nursing*, 24(1): 26–33.

Catford, J. (2005) 'The Bangkok Conference: Steering Countries to Build National Capacity for Health Promotion', *Health Promotion International*, 20: 1–6.

Davey, B. (2005) 'Key Global Health Concerns for the Twenty-first Century', in Scriven, A. and Garman, S. (eds), *Promoting Health: Global Perspectives* (Basingstoke: Palgrave Macmillan): 19–32.

DoH (2004) *Policy Appraisal and Health* (London: DoH).

Drager, N. and Fidler, D. (2007) 'Foreign Policy, Trade and Health: At the Cutting Edge of Global Diplomacy', *Bulletin of the World Health Organization*, 85(3): 162.

Horne, M. (2003) 'Identifying the Health Needs of Communities and Populations', in Costello, J. and Haggart, M. (eds), *Public Health and Society* (Basingstoke: Palgrave Macmillan): 119–3.

Hosseinpoor, A.R., Van Doorslaer, E., Speybroeck, N., Naghavi, M., Mohammad, K., Delavar, B., Jamshidi, H. and Vega, J. (2006) 'Decomposing Socioeconomic Inequality in Mortality in Iran', *International Journal of Epidemiology*, 35: 1211–19.

Jenkins, R. (2004) 'Globalization, Production, Employment and Poverty: Debates and Evidence', *Journal of International Development*, 16: 1–12.

Levin, L.S. and Ziglio, E. (2003) 'Health Promotion as an Investment Strategy: A Perspective for the Twenty-first Century', in Sidell, M., Jones, L., Katz, J., Peberdy, A. and Douglas, J. (eds), *Debates and Dilemmas in Promoting Health: A Reader*, 2nd edn (Basingstoke: Palgrave): 412–22.

Magnusson, R.S. (2007) 'Non-communicable Diseases and Global Health Governance: Enhancing Global Processes to Improve Health Development', *Globalization and Health*, 3(2): 1–16. Available online at http://www.globalizationandhealth.com/content/3/1/2 (accessed 25 November 2008).

Mathers, C.D. and Loncar, D. (2006) 'Projections of Global Mortality and Burden of Disease from 2002 to 2030', *PLoS Med*, 3, (11): e442, doi:10.1371.journal.pmed.0030442.

McDaid, D. and Oliver, A. (2005) 'Inequalities in Health: International Patterns and Trends', in Scriven, A. and Garman, S. (eds), *Promoting Health: Global Perspectives* (Basingstoke: Palgrave Macmillan): 33–47.

McKeown, T. (1976) *The Modern Rise of Population* (New York: Academic Press).

McKeown, T. (1979) *The Role of Medicine: Dream, Mirage or Nemesis?* (Oxford: Basil Blackwell).

McMichael, A.J. and Beaglehole, R. (2003) 'The Changing Global Context of Public Health', in Sidell, M., Jones, L., Katz, J., Peberdy, A. and Douglas, J. (eds), *Debates and Dilemmas in Promoting Health: A Reader*, 2nd edn (Basingstoke: Palgrave): 211–20.

Mittelmark, M. (2005) 'Global Health Promotion: Challenges and Opportunities', in Scriven, A. and Garman, S. (eds), *Promoting Health: Global Perspectives* (Basingstoke: Palgrave Macmillan): 48–57.

Peersman, G. (2001) 'Promoting Health: Principles of Practice and Evaluation', in Oliver, S. and Peersman, G. (eds), *Using Research for Effective Health Promotion* (Buckingham: Open University Press): 3–15.

Sargent, R.P., Shepard, R.M. and Glantz, S.A. (2004) 'Reduced Incidence of Admissions for Myocardial Infarction associated with Public Smoking Ban: Before and After Study', *BMJ*, 328(7446): 977–80.

Scriven, A. (2005) 'Promoting Health: A Global Context and Rationale', in Scriven, A. and Garman, S. (eds), *Promoting Health: Global Perspectives* (Basingstoke: Palgrave Macmillan): 1–13.

Tones, K. and Tilford, S. (2001) *Health Promotion: Effectiveness, Efficiency and Equity*, 3rd edn (Cheltenham: Nelson Thornes).

UN (2007) *The Millennium Development Goals Report* (New York: United Nations).

UN General Assembly (2000) *United Nations Millennium Declaration*. Available online: http://www.un.org/millennium/declaration/ares552e.htm (accessed 25 November 2008).

UNAIDS/WHO (2006) *AIDS Epidemic Update*, Joint United Nations Programme on HIV/AIDS, UNAIDS/06.29E (Geneva: WHO).

WHO (1978) *Declaration of Alma-Ata* (Geneva: WHO).

WHO (1986) *Ottawa Charter for Health Promotion* (Geneva: WHO).

WHO (2003) *Diet, Nutrition and the Prevention of Chronic Diseases* (Geneva: WHO). Available online at http://www.who.int/hpr/NPH/docs/who_fao_expert_report.pdf

WHO (2005) *The Bangkok Charter for Health Promotion in a Globalized World* (Geneva: WHO).

WHO (2006) *Preventing Disease Through Healthy Environments: Towards an Estimate of the Environmental Burden of Disease* (Geneva: WHO).

WHO (2007a) *The World Health Report 2007: A Safer Future: Global Public Health Security in the 21st Century* (Geneva: WHO).

WHO (2007b) *World Health Statistics 2007* (Geneva: WHO).

WHO (2007c) *Protection from Exposure to Second-hand Tobacco Smoke: Policy Recommendations* (Geneva: WHO).

Whitehead, D. (2009) 'Reconciling the Differences between Health Promotion in Nursing and "General" Health Promotion: A Discussion Paper', *International Journal of Nursing Studies*, 46(6): 865–74.

Yach, D., Beaglehole, R. and Hawkes, C. (2005) 'Globalisation and Noncommunicable Diseases', in Scriven, A. and Garman, S. (eds), *Promoting Health: Global Perspectives* (Basingstoke: Palgrave Macmillan): 77–89.

Answers to Tutorial Briefs

1 Contextualizing health promotion

Tutorial brief 1.1

No single answer can be given here. Your perception of health is likely to be highly personal. The things that allow you to consider yourself as healthy might include:

- The absence of disease
- The fulfilment of basic needs (such as food, water, shelter)
- The ability to socialize with others
- The ability to respond to everyday demands
- Physical fitness
- The ability to make decisions about your life

Tutorial brief 1.2

- You might have *power over* your client group because you have access to resources and information that affect their health and you might be making decisions about their health.
- This might have a disempowering effect if you do not involve your group in decision-making and could lead to a top-down, authoritarian approach to health promotion.
- Your managers and colleagues might have *power over* you because they make decisions that affect the way that you practice.
- Again, if you and your client groups are not able to influence or contribute to these decisions, this will have a disempowering effect that confines any intervention to an individual and authoritarian strategy.
- You might have *power with* your clients because you are able to discuss issues with them and facilitate them in identifying problems, making decisions and resolving issues, independently or collectively.
- This will help to empower your client group because they will be actively engaged in all aspects of the interventions, leading to a collective and negotiated strategy.

Tutorial brief 1.3

1   Information-giving

Strengths:

- Can result in improved knowledge of threats to health from risky behaviour
- Is advocated in many policy documents

Limitations:

- Can lead to victim-blaming
- Has little effect on the health of the general population

2   Self-empowerment

Strengths:

- Leads to improved self-esteem, self-confidence and increased health-related skills

Limitations:

- Has little effect on the health of the whole population
- Motives of professionals can be dubious
- Disempowered professionals might not be able to facilitate the empowerment of their clients

3   Behaviour change

Strengths:

- Clear links exist between lifestyle and health

Limitations:

- Effectiveness of approach is often limited
- Can lead to victim-blaming
- Has little effect on the health of the general population

Tutorial brief 1.4

No single answer can be given here. Your goals will depend on the focus of your intervention. The sort of outcomes that you could expect would be:

- Improved understanding of the causes of illness
- Improved understanding of the link between lifestyles and ill health

- Raised awareness of health issues
- Increase self-esteem
- Improved self-efficacy
- Enhanced assertiveness and negotiation skills
- Self-empowerment
- Attitude change
- Change in behaviour

Tutorial brief 1.5

No single answer can be given here. The things that need to put in place will depend on the intervention that you are planning. It might include:

- A sound understanding of the community developed through strategies such as community needs assessments and health impact assessments
- Long-term commitment from the community to include:
  - Ownership of the issue by the community
  - Identification of the key people who will be involved in the initiative
  - Identification of the roles that people will assume
  - Agreement on the goals of the initiative
- The resources that will be needed for the activity, such as:
  - Venue
  - Financial resources
  - Equipment
  - Crèche facilities
  - Professionals from various disciplines
  - Training for community members who wish to participate

2 Health promotion theory, models and approaches

Tutorial brief 2.1

You might wish to return to the discussion in Chapter 1 to refresh yourself about definitions of health education and health promotion. There are no right or wrong answers with regard to what you might identify as health promotion within your own practice. It might be that your ideas about health promotion change and/or evolve as you engage with the contents of this textbook.

Tutorial brief 2.2

There is no right or wrong answer to this question, but it should have provided you with an opportunity to reflect more critically on your practice, and help identify the ways in which you work in terms of top-down versus bottom-up approaches.

Tutorial brief 2.3

There is no right or wrong answer to this question, but it should have provided you with an opportunity to reflect more critically on your practice and the approaches that you might use in terms of Naidoo and Wills' framework.

Tutorial brief 2.4

Again, there is no right or wrong answer here. Whether or not you agree or disagree with Sykes's point of view is dependent on your perspective. However, it is good discipline to be able to defend your point of view, providing evidence to support it.

Tutorial brief 2.5

You will probably have come up with a useful list for this tutorial brief. Naidoo and Wills (2000) provide a good exploration of the advantages and disadvantages of using the community development approach. The following information is adapted from their work:

Advantages of the community development approach:

- It might be more likely to gain people's support, since it starts with them and the situations in which they find themselves
- It focuses on what causes ill health, rather than the symptoms of it
- It can produce awareness of the social causes of ill health
- The process can be enabling and build confidence
- It can encourage the building of skills (transferable skills – such as communication skills, for example)
- The health promoter and the members of the community should be able to work together as equal partners

Disadvantages of the community development approach:

- It can take a great deal of time
- It is often difficult to prove that it has worked (hard to measure and evaluate)
- It might produce contradiction or conflict for the health promoter in terms of to whom they feel answerable (their employer, the funder or the community itself)
- It usually involves only small groups of people
- It might draw attention away from the wider issues by focusing on specific neighbourhoods or communities

3 Health promotion and the role and function of the nurse

There can be no standard answers to any of the tutorial brief exercises in this chapter. They are all asking the reader to draw on personal experiences and constructs. Therefore, the answers are personal in themselves.

4 A systematic approach to health promotion

Tutorial brief 4.1

No single answer can be given here. You will find some theoretical models useful and others not – whether that is parts of them or the models as a whole.

Tutorial brief 4.2

When assessing a community, a range of information must be gathered for effective assessment and programming. The list below is taken from the bulleted lists in the text in the assessment section of this chapter.

- History of the community – both past and recent
- General environment
- Nature of residents
- Types of organization
- Communication methods and structures
- Where the seats of power and leadership lay
- Listening to, and taking notice of, the community
- Assessing local social and economic indicators
- Drawing upon epidemiological data – but also realizing its limitations, and so striving for broader approaches to health assessment
- Seeking the views of health professionals and other professionals who work within the assessed community
- Reviewing state, regional or national policies – especially those emerging from community consultation
- Generally observing and measuring 'the lay of the land'
- Mapping resources
- Identifying players who could/will help and assist
- Identifying structural factors already in place – that is, human resources, health systems, gate-keepers, locations and so on
- Performing a current strengths, weaknesses, opportunities and threats (SWOT) analysis of the community and its people

Tutorial brief 4.3

On the subject of the different categories of community need:

- *Felt need* is a subjective need based on what people say that they feel that they need for their health. This form of need is useful for identifying local issues as they pertain to small groups, and allows individuals to feel that they are part of the assessment process.
- *Expressed need* is more about need based on demand. It goes beyond felt need to the basis of actioning by making felt need more 'concrete'. Demand for new services or support for existing health related services is an example.
- *Normative need* is need based on professional opinion or research and/or evidence based activity. It is an objective need that is more determined by experts and is therefore more likely to be governed by nurses rather than lay community members – unless those lay community members are deemed experts in their own right. Health promotion, based on normative need alone, is likely to be alienating to the community at large.
- *Comparative need* is based on comparing services within one geographical area with those of another similar area of demographic. Such information provides compelling evidence for claiming resources for services where they are lacking in one demographic and not in others.

Tutorial brief 4.4

Your list might include factors such as:

- Education
- Leisure and recreation facilities
- Lifestyle
- Levels of crime assessed against policing and justice systems
- Communications and media
- Social systems
- Environment
- Transportation
- Economic wealth
- Welfare
- Access to and availability of health services
- Values, attitudes, beliefs, culture, religion and language
- Population demographics – age, gender
- Safety issues
- Utilities and services
- Business and labour markets

Tutorial brief 4.5

Your list might include factors such as:

- Ensuring that original assessed and planned activities and time frames are being adhered to
- Ensuring that due process is being followed, that effective communication on progress between stakeholders is in evidence, and that any issues, barriers and dilemmas are reported and acted on accordingly
- Ensuring a series of mini-reviews and evaluations are taking place
- Ensuring that nurses and other health professionals monitor progress, act on presented issues, and change the course of any intervention where necessary
- Ensuring flexibility against unanticipated outcomes

Tutorial brief 4.6

Your list might include factors such as:

- Positive feedback from key stakeholders in the community
- Positive feedback from the general lay community
- Positive epidemiological data – that is, changes in mortality/morbidity rates
- Programme is cost-effective and cost-efficient
- New and better health services infrastructure
- More visible health services infrastructure
- Equitable access for all community residents to health services
- Those most in need have been specifically targeted
- Improved health education
- Targeted health media campaigns
- Visible political and health policy representation
- The 4 Es: effectiveness, efficiency, efficacy and equity

Tutorial brief 4.7

For many, in and outside of health promotion circles, 'quality' evidence comes in the form of generalizable experimental research. However, for health promotion programmes this is not always available or appropriate. Other forms of evidence might include:

- Results from non-experimental quantitative studies – for example, surveys
- Results of qualitative research studies
- Local, national and international policies and documents
- Health services data and audit

- Professional experience and opinion
- Lay community experience and opinion
- Your own experience and opinion
- Press and media reports

5 Settings-based health promotion

Tutorial brief 5.1

No single answer can be given here. Your individual and group perceptions and experiences will determine the extent to which you answer this question about health-promoting hospitals.

Tutorial brief 5.2

Positive factors:

- Targeting children at a young age can results in positive life-long health practices
- Children can be more receptive to positive messages than their older counterparts
- School compliance systems mean that children might be more likely to adopt what they are taught
- Health promotion can be 'hands-on' and experiential within the classroom and field setting

Negative factors:

- Health-promoting factors at school might not transfer to a child's home setting or be supported by other family members
- Busy lifestyles and media influence might mean unhealthy options are the most convenient – that is, processed foods
- It might be difficult to implement health promotion in an already 'crammed' national curriculum
- Negative influences, such as peer pressure and bullying, might negate positive health promotion activities
- Not all schools are equal – in terms of their geography, resources, infrastructure and social position of children

Tutorial brief 5.3

1. No single answer can be given here. Your individual and group perceptions and experiences will determine the extent to which you answer this question about

your work-related health conditions and status. It is generally known, however, that organizational, educational and management issues are the main influences on health professionals' health-related practices. For many, the same issue could be either positive or negative – or a mixture of both. For example, you might work within an open, collegial, common goal team-working environment – or you might work in a far less functional, progressive and rewarding environment.

2. Again, no single answer can be given here. Your already identified negative factors will determine the extent of what reforms need to be in place. What would be useful, as part of this exercise, is to identify the factors that are beyond your control (although some might argue that all issues are within the control of those who encounter them) and those that you can influence directly. For those that you can influence, think about how you could begin to implement them now.

6 Evidence-based practice in health promotion

Tutorial brief 6.1

Identify the strengths and limitations of involving lay advisors in defining the approach of a smoking cessation service?

Some possible suggestions:
Pros:

- Local people with local knowledge
- Able to understand context – such as social class, ethnic group
- Taps into lay knowledge (that is, 'everyday reality')
- Professional might be perceived as threatening, lay advisor seen as a peer
- Less likely to use medical jargon

Cons:

- Might lack certain professional knowledge (for example, medical or pharmacological)
- Could be too focused on their own personal experience

Tutorial brief 6.2

What are the pros and cons of using community indicators rather than traditional epidemiological data (such as teenage pregnancy rates) as evidence of the success, or otherwise, of a health promotion intervention?

Epidemiological data (such as mortality and morbidity rates) are useful. Nevertheless, for communities, numerical data can appear distant from people's personal experience. Also, whilst interventions might affect rates, this might take some time to be reflected in the epidemiological figures. Community indicators are usually defined (and therefore owned) by the community members themselves, suggesting a common goal. Community indicators can be measures of well-being or quality of life (that is, a positive measure), rather than of levels of illness or disability. They often reflect the values of that particular community and are usually more immediate.

Tutorial brief 6.3

Given the barriers in implementing evidence-based health promotion identified above, what solutions can you suggest to overcome these?

- Continuing professional development in research utilization skills, including searching literature and critical appraisal
- Development of partnerships between health-promoters and academics – for example, 'ground rounds' or research discussion groups
- Health-promoters to be required to present the evidence base for their proposed health promotion intervention before it is given the go ahead by managers
- Development of networks of practitioners with similar interests: several organizations, such as the Royal College of Nursing and the United Kingdom Public Health Alliance (UKPHA) have special interest groups that focus on particular populations or issues – for example, homeless people or food poverty
- Maintain a widescreen view of what counts as evidence
- Disseminate findings of evaluation of interventions, even if they did not meet their original planned outcomes, at conferences, in journals and so on
- Authors and journal editors work to maximize clarity of implications for practice of articles

7 Health promotion – politics, policy and ethics

Tutorial brief 7.1

What are the ethical considerations behind such a technique (as harm reduction) if it appears to condone an illegal behaviour?

- Should nurses judge the behaviour of their patients, or is their duty to provide care for everyone on a non-discriminatory basis?
- The HIV pandemic caused clinicians in many countries to change their views about the balance of public protection. With no cure for HIV/AIDS and only

prevention as a means of limiting the spread of the infection, a different approach was needed to help vulnerable groups such as injecting drug users, men who have sex with men, and sex workers. If clinicians cannot persuade individuals to end high-risk behaviour completely, then harm reduction techniques might minimize the harm to individuals and the population at large.

- What is the difference, ethically, between providing health promotion for someone convicted of a crime and in prison, and someone who is an illicit drug user in the community?

Tutorial brief 7.2

Consider the importance of generating a sound evidence base to support health promotion practice. How can this evidence base be used to influence the opinion of politicians and local communities?

- People's opinion can be influenced by a wide range of factors, including many that are subjective – for example, personal experience, articles in newspapers and religious belief
- Such opinions might influence the views of communities and community groups about what might make a difference to their health
- Sound evidence is difficult to contradict, or be twisted to suit political opinion
- Sound evidence can be utilized to brief the media and, in turn, influence opinion

Tutorial brief 7.3

Why should the World Health Organization be reluctant to take an official position on sexual health, having convened an international group to develop these definitions?

- Sexual health promotion for children and young people is a contentious issue for some communities and has been the subject of court cases regarding the balance of rights between parents and young people.
- In some countries, cultures and religions, men having sexual intercourse with men, and women who have sex for money are perceived as committing moral and/or criminal offences.
- The World Health Organization needs to be able work in many countries including nations/cultures that have the views outlined above, therefore a diplomatic stance might be needed to enable any health promotion to be carried out.
- The World Health Organization is also dependant on countries and charitable organizations for the funding it needs to carry out its public health programmes. Offending such donors would limit its ability to carry out its health promotion activity.

Tutorial brief 7.4

What evidence is there to suggest that Western based organizations have tried to influence the public health policy of African states?

- High profile events such as Band Aid, Live Aid and Red Nose Day are just some examples of Western intervention in Africa. The funds raised are used for projects such as HIV prevention and related sexual health programmes.
- Benefactors, such as Bill Gates of 'Microsoft' fame, have also donated large sums of money to projects in Africa.
- Christian faith based organizations have also supported aid programmes in Africa, making funds available to impoverished communities.

Tutorial brief 7.5

How much should external agencies be able to influence the health promotion programmes they fund? Should the concept of 'he who pays the piper calls the tune' apply? What if the funding body is a commercial company: does that alter the situation?

- Health promotion is often seen as an easy area in which to make cuts when health service resources are under pressure. This factor might influence nurses to accept funding from other sources. Such finances might include charitable sources and from commercial sources such as drug companies. Nurses might view these two funding sources as ethically different, since charitable monies have been raised for benevolent reasons whereas commercial organizations seek to make a profit from their products.
- What ethical constraints should practitioners consider when seeking or accepting funding from any organization? Can there be an ethical relationship with a company that makes a profit from the products that its sells? Some commercial companies have set aside part of their profits into charitable trusts. Does this factor change the ethical considerations regarding use of this source of funding?
- The UK government has formed a charitable trust with the alcoholic drinks industry known as the 'Drink Aware Trust'. This charity's aim is to promote harm reduction messages regarding alcohol use. The government earns significant funding from tax revenue from the sale of alcohol. The alcohol industry directly and indirectly employs large numbers of people in hotels, pubs, clubs, brewing, tourism and so on, and therefore contributes further taxes to the government. Alcohol misuse has been identified as a common reason for individuals indulging in risky sexual behaviour.

Tutorial brief 7.6

What factors might have influenced the local and national governments to take differing positions on the issue of street sex working?

- National and local politics can have different factors influencing them. This might mean that politicians from the same political party can have opposing views on the same issue, as they are viewing it from different perspectives. These factors can include religion and culture, but can also include economic and social issues. The effects on house prices, business viability and urban renewal can also be a consideration.
- In the case of Liverpool, a major consultation exercise had demonstrated a strong consensus for a new approach to addressing street prostitution. The murder in the city of two young women who were sex workers appeared to have influenced local opinion towards this different approach. The mothers of these young women have also played a significant part in influencing local opinion, as they supported the proposals for a managed zone.
- The murder of five sex workers in Ipswich has re-opened the debate in the UK about the government's strategy.
- In the UK, the main political parties believe that they must be seen to be 'tough on crime', therefore a policy on prostitution that appears to be 'soft on crime' will damage the reputation of the party that proposes it.
- In Australia and New Zealand, national and state governments have adopted similar pragmatic harm reduction policies as those in Holland and Germany, with decriminalization of sex-workers. This approach has enabled nurses and other health professionals to carry out health promotion programmes within a more positive and liberal political environment.

8 Current and future developments in health promotion

Tutorial brief 8.1

Your list might have had a biomedical slant and included factors such as:

- Technological advances
- Development of antibiotic therapy and other medicines
- Immunization programmes
- Better health screening
- Development on anaesthesia
- Improved maternal and child care
- Advances in surgical and medical knowledge/procedures

Or, your list might have had more of an environmental/social focus such as:

- Improved nutrition
- Better hygiene
- Availability of contraception
- Improved sanitation
- Better housing
- Wider access to education
- Improved access to healthcare

As discussed in the chapter, there are a number of factors associated with declining death rates, and all of the points included in the lists have played a significant part.

Tutorial brief 8.2

There are many things that you might have listed. Your answer might look something like this:

Improvements in health	Declines in health
• We no longer suffer from diseases such as cholera	• New diseases have emerged such as HIV/AIDS, avian influenza
• We have better living conditions	• Certain bacteria have become resistant to antibiotics – for example, MRSA
• We are better educated about health	• People are living longer and suffering from diseases of old age – such as arthritis, cataracts, heart disease
• We have technology and the media to provide positive information on health	
• We enjoy better social lives	• Homelessness is a problem
• Working conditions have improved	• Many people in society are marginalized and suffer stigmatization
• We have better hygiene	
• Legislation helps to protect us – for example, seat belt laws, smoking bans	• The media and communication technology, such as the Internet, can promote unhealthy lifestyles
• Women have more rights	
• We are more tolerant of people being different to ourselves	• Social pressures to conform to certain body sizes have lead to diseases such as anorexia nervosa and bulimia
• Globalization means peopl.e are able to travel to work and live in other countries – sometimes to avoid oppression in their country of origin	
• Better financial security	• Peoples diets are higher in fat and salt
• People live longer work and home life is challenging	• Some food produce might be harmful to health – for example, additives, GM food
• Cancer survival rates have improved	• People live an increasingly sedentary lifestyle
• Most of us have good access to healthcare	• Alcohol consumption has increased, particularly in women and youths
• Infant mortality has decreased	

and strokes are rising

- Infections can be treated
- Improved screening means conditions can be treated early
- Advances in genetics make the avoidance of pollution has caused increases in conditions as asthma
- People have access to a varied diet
- People take preventative measures against sexually transmitted diseases
- People are aware of dangers such as sun exposure

- People suffer from high levels of stress
- Balancing modern day stresses such as
- Smoking and drug taking have increased
- Obesity rates are increasing
- Conditions such as coronary heart disease
- Many people are socially isolated, particularly older people
- Inequalities in health have increased
- Increased pollution has caused increases in such as asthma

Note: Some things might be included in both lists. For example, better financial security can bring about better living conditions and access to essential resources such as food. However, increased wealth and associated food abundance also have potential to lead to problems of obesity.

Tutorial brief 8.3

Globalization can positively affect health by providing the opportunity for sharing of experiences across countries. It means that there are opportunities for cooperation across the globe to enable countries to learn from one another and to work collaboratively to reduce transnational risks.

Globalization can have a negative influence on health by eroding environmental conditions and through the 'spread' of non-communicable diseases across the globe, particularly to developing countries. Additionally, the increased mobility of the world's population (a feature of globalization) has made the spread of diseases such as severe acute respiratory syndrome (SARS) and avian influenza a major global health concern.

Tutorial brief 8.4

In the same way that health has become a global issue, nursing, too, has to take on a global perspective. It is important that individual nurses see their part in this process. They need to look beyond their own countries and stay attuned to international aspects of nursing. They can achieve this by accessing global policies and reading international literature, for example. Accessing the above can facilitate their awareness of positive developments and advances in health care in countries other than their own. It can also alert them to challenges to health arising in another part of the world. Both of these things are important because the effects of globalization are such that developments in one part of the world (either positive or negative) are likely to affect health and nursing in other parts of the world at some point.

Tutorial brief 8.5

Nursing can achieve a great deal. It has the strength of a significant global workforce in terms of numbers. It can respond to changing health needs and develop new technologies, systems and policies to promote health. However, because health is determined by a complex interplay of social, demographic, economic and environmental factors, health promotion cannot be achieved by nursing and the health sector alone. It requires a commitment to work together across different sectors.

Tutorial brief 8.6

It is not necessary to try to commit the targets associated with the millennium development goals to memory; however, being aware of their existence is important. Once you have retrieved and saved a copy, you can access them as appropriate to your needs.

Index